WHY LIVING A SIMPLE LIFE IS BETTER FOR YOU

RACHEL STONE

Hackney and Jones

HACKNEY & JONES

Claim Your Freebie NOW!

Get Good At Problem Solving

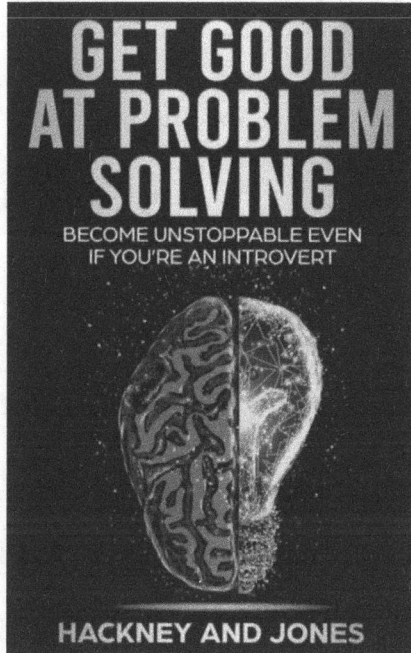

Want to know the secret behind getting good at problem solving? Everyone seems to be able to do it, but you're stuck in the pile of endless to-do lists with little progress.

Ok, so how do I get my FREE book?

EASY! See the next page

Claim Your Freebie NOW

Instructions:

1. Open the camera or the QR reader application on your smartphone.

2. Point your camera at the QR code to scan the QR code.

3. A notification will pop-up on screen.

4. Click on the notification to open the website link

SCAN ME

Also By Rachel Stone

How To Remove Negativity From Your Life

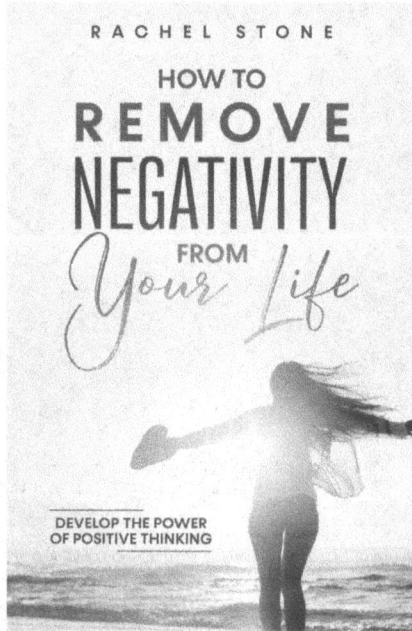

Rid yourself forever from the negative thoughts that plague your life with this amazing, life-changing book.

Also By Rachel Stone

Start Being Fearless, Stop Being Scared

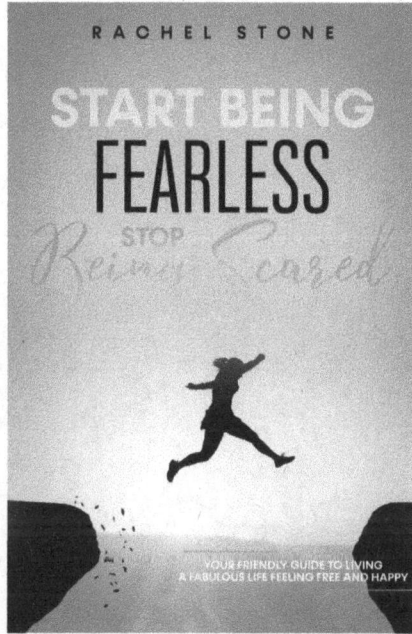

Fed up of being scared of the things in life that hold you back? It's time to take control back and start being fearless.

Also By Rachel Stone

How To Heal Toxic Thoughts

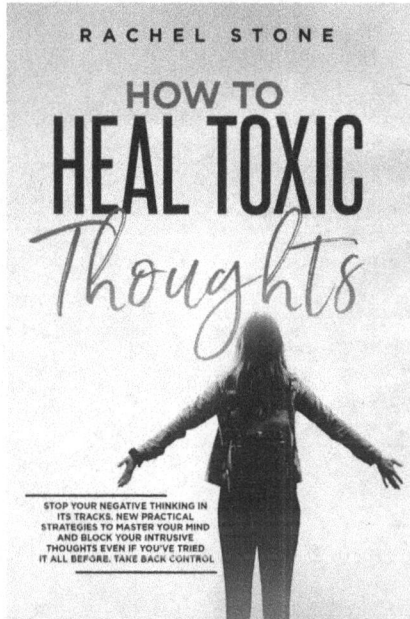

Are you sick of your whole day being ruined due to your overthinking? Have you had enough of self-sabotaging everything good in your life? Do you want practical strategies to finally have a peaceful night's sleep?

Grab the Rachel Stone series NOW

Instructions:

1. Open the camera or the QR reader application on your smartphone.

2. Point your camera at the QR code to scan the QR code.

3. A notification will pop-up on screen.

4. Click on the notification to open the website link

SCAN ME

Introduction

It is said that *when the student is ready, the teacher will appear.* If you're reading this, you're ready to take the next step in your personal growth. You are ready to start consciously generating and getting more of what you truly desire in your life.

What if I told you that having fewer things could make you happier? Doesn't it sound a little crazy? That's because we are bombarded with signals to the contrary every day and wherever we turn:

- Purchase this, and you'll be prettier.
- Own this, and you'll be more successful.
- Own this, and your happiness will know no boundaries.

We've purchased this, that, and the other item. So we must be in seventh heaven. For the large majority of us, the answer is "no." In reality, quite often, the opposite is true: many of these goods, and their false promises, steadily drain the money from our pockets, the magic from our relationships, and the joy from our lives. Have you ever looked around your house at all the stuff you've purchased, inherited, or been given and felt overwhelmed rather than over-joyed? Do you have credit card debt and can't remember the purchases for which you're making payments? Do you privately wish a gale force wind would blow the clutter out of your home, giving you a chance to start over? If this is the case, a simple lifestyle might be your salvation.

To begin, let us define the term "minimalism." As it's typically linked with stylish, multimillion-dollar apartments with three pieces of furniture, it appears to have acquired a rather intimidating, elitist aspect. The term brings up thoughts of minimalist rooms, concrete flooring, and shining white surfaces. It all sounds extremely serious, sober, and sterile. What function could it possibly play in the lives of people who have children, pets, hobbies, junk mail, and laundry?

When most people hear the word "minimalism," they think "empty." Unfortunately, the word "empty" isn't particularly attractive; it's often linked with loss, deprivation, and scarcity. But consider "empty" from a different perspective—think about what it is rather than what it isn't—and you have "space." Space! That is something we could all benefit from more of! Space in our closets, garages, schedules, space to think, play, create, and enjoy ourselves with our families...that is the beauty of minimalism.

Consider this: a container is most useful when it is empty. We can't enjoy fresh coffee if the grounds are old, and we can't show off our garden's blooms if the vase is full of wilted flowers. Similarly, when our homes—the containers of our everyday lives—are cluttered, our souls take a back seat to our possessions. We no longer have the time, energy, or room to try new things. We feel suffocated and restricted as if we can't completely stretch out and express ourselves.

We get control of our belongings by becoming minimalists. We reclaim our space and bring function and possibility back into our houses. We remake our homes to make them open, airy, and sensitive to the substance of our lives. We announce our freedom from the tyranny of clutter. It's positively free!

That's fantastic, but how do we get there? Where do we begin? What differentiates this book from all the other books on life organisation?

Unlike other organising books, this one isn't about buying fancy containers or storage systems to shuffle about your belongings;

rather, it's about reducing the amount of stuff you have to deal with. Furthermore, you will not be required to complete tests, checklists, or charts—who has time for that? And there will be no thousands of case studies on other people's trash; the emphasis here is on you.

We'll begin by developing a minimalist attitude. Don't worry; it's not difficult! We'll think about the joys and benefits of living a clutter-free life; it'll give us the drive we need later while dealing with grandma's old china. We'll learn to recognise our possessions for what they are, therefore weakening whatever influence they may have over us, and we'll find the freedom of living with just "enough" to fulfil our requirements. We'll even get philosophical about how our new minimalism will improve our lives and affect positive change in the world.

What's the big deal? Because decluttering is similar to dieting. We may go right in, count our belongings like calories, and "starve" ourselves for quick results. All too frequently, though, we will feel starved, go on a binge, and then find ourselves right back where we started. First, we must change our thoughts and habits, much like moving from a meat-and-potatoes to a Mediterranean diet. Developing a minimalist mindset will change how we think about the things we own and the things we bring into our lives. Instead of a quick cure, it will be a long-term commitment to a new and delightful way of life.

Each room in the house has its own set of problems. As a result, we'll go room by room, investigating more detailed approaches to each one. We'll begin in the family room, transforming it into a versatile, lively area for us to enjoy our leisure activities. We'll discuss the pros and cons of each piece of furniture, as well as what to do with all of those books, DVDs, video games, and art supplies. Then we'll go to the bedroom, where we'll remove the excess to create a tranquil haven for our tired spirits. Our objective is to create a clear, peaceful, and uncluttered place that calms and rejuvenates us.

We'll devote a whole chapter to clothing concerns because so many of us have overcrowded closets. (If you follow the suggestions within, you'll look fantastic in a fraction of your present outfits.) Once we've gotten into a rhythm, we'll target the mountains of papers in our home offices, reducing the flow into our inboxes from a torrent to a trickle. Our minimalist makeover will tame even the messiest workstations!

Finally, we'll look at how being a minimalist helps us be better citizens of the Earth and protect its richness for future generations. We'll examine the actual effect of our purchasing decisions, analysing both the human and environmental costs of the items we buy, and discover the far-reaching advantages of living lightly and gracefully on the Earth. The greatest part: we'll learn how to save space in our closets while also helping the world.

Are you ready to get rid of the clutter once and for all? Simply turn the page for your first dose of minimalist philosophy; in a matter of minutes, you'll be on your way to a simpler, more stream-lined, and more peaceful life.

1

What Exactly Do We Mean By
"A Simple Life"?

A SIMPLE LIFE is devoid of excess, overconsumption, and material possessions. It entails a variety of voluntary activities aimed towards enhancing one's assets and self-sufficiency. It is distinguished by a culture of abstaining from luxury, emphasising needs rather than wants.

A simple life is uncomplicated, uncluttered, and full of contentment. Peaceful. Living a simple life entails getting rid of anything that does not provide value to your life. The next question is, "What is valuable to you?" The solutions are as unique as you are, but you should give this one some serious thought. We frequently believe that stuff has worth it because of the cost to our lives. This is not correct. The price tag does not always correspond to the value or usefulness. Frequently, the very things we strive for become onerous once we have them.

If you genuinely want to live a simple life, you must confront the reality of your existing way of living. You'll have to answer some difficult questions. Then you must be driven to make adjustments that are compatible with your new 'truths.' Are you ready?

Do You Understand What Stress Is?

On a Saturday afternoon, I drove to a highly busy shopping area to ask the first 100 people I saw three questions and then evaluated their responses.

The first question was, "Do you understand what stress is?" Ninety-nine people said "yes," with the hundredth too busy shopping to react! "What is stress?" was the second question. The 99 persons I interviewed said that stress was caused by "time pressure"—people get anxious when they do not have enough time to complete what they want to do in the time they have. The final question asked, "Which group do you believe is the most stressed: the elderly, children, or adults?" The 99 blithely replied, "No question! Adults!"

This is a reasonable response. Adults are the most stressed group if stress is a result of time pressure, given the pressure of schedules, the 100,000 jobs to do, children to take to and from daycare, the never-ending work, children's sports activities in the evenings and on weekends, ageing parents who need assistance, and the list goes on!

Why do these folks believe that the elderly and children are less stressed than they are? It's because their notion of stress centres around time constraints. Because older adults are retired, they have all the time they desire. Therefore time constraints cannot be a source of worry for them. Furthermore, we frequently caricature the elderly: they move slowly, drive slowly, and do everything slowly. As a result, they cannot be under time restrictions and, as a result, cannot be more stressed than we are.

Similarly, our children do not appear to be pressed for time. They do not have an oppressive employer, urgent bills to pay at the end of the month, or frantic shopping to complete; all they have to do is spend time with their friends and engage in their favourite hobbies. As a result, they would not be stressed.

The first misconception in the general view of stress is that because stress results from time constraints, we assume that the elderly and children are inherently less worried than adults. This is incorrect.

Scientific findings during the previous two decades demonstrate that the contrary is true. Stress has a far greater impact on their brains than it does on ours. The elderly and children are significantly more sensitive to stress than adults. Indeed, this susceptibility rises among the elderly due to the influence stress has on ageing and progressively deteriorating brain—it has been demonstrated that stress has the power to accelerate the ageing of the brain in the elderly.

Because their brains are still developing, children's brains are more sensitive to stress. Stress has also been found to slow the development of some areas or functions of the brain in children.

Along with the myth of time pressure as a source of stress, a new version has emerged in recent years, this time involving children. According to this notion, parents continuously urge their children to rush through various activities such as going to school, doing homework, and participating in one sport or extracurricular activity after another, both during the week and on the weekends. As a result, parents place time constraints on their children. This is frequently repeated in newspapers and publications, implying that the numerous sports and cultural activities in which our kids are enrolled in the evenings and on weekends lead them to rush and so have become a source of stress. Because stress is associated with time constraints, the connection is obvious: children, like adults, are stressed.

In addition to dealing with their stress, impoverished parents must now evaluate if including their children in sports activities may cause them stress, given the continuous message that exercise is the key to preventing childhood obesity. "It's insane. Either we stress our children out, or they get obese!"

But is it truly time pressure that causes stress in our children? Children are energetic, and sports frequently replace the distance that children in a previous period would have walked to school. Not only do kids no longer walk to school, but video games have become an important part of their daily lives. So, before assuming that sports activities stress children because they create time pressure, consider if the tension is truly caused by time pressure. I confidently state that it is not!

3

Time Pressure Is Not The Same As Stress

Allow me to dispel the first myth about stress before enrolling your child for the next hockey camp. Time constraints do not cause stress. Let us look at the evidence to the contrary.

If stress is only the product of time constraints, how can we be stressed during a visit to the dentist on a day off? In this scenario, you will agree that time is irrelevant because you are not working. And the receptionist or dental hygienist will not rush you to the dentist's chair with a stopwatch in hand! However, the ordinary individual feels agitated by a visit to the dentist, and the tension is much relieved upon leaving the dentist's office, even if the cost is large.

Consider the following instances. What about the immense tension you feel when you or someone you care about is diagnosed with a serious illness? Or when you're summoned to the boss's office during a major corporate reorganisation? Or when your mother-in-law comes up on a Friday night and reveals that she's coming to stay the weekend, after you've been looking forward to a relaxing few days all week? In terms of time pressure, how do we explain stress in these situations?

I'm sure you'll feel a spike of tension in all of these scenarios, at least as strong as if you were late picking up the kids from daycare. However, there is no time constraint in any of these cases. As a consequence, stress is not caused by a lack of time. But what exactly is it that creates stress? The most comprehensive approach to address this issue would be to go back in time and examine how the notion of stress arose, how it has evolved through time, and how scientists view it now.

I know you're eager to get to the meat of the matter and learn more about what causes a stress reaction. That is why I won't bore you with a lengthy chapter on the history of stress science.

Researchers have discovered that our subjective pressure does not cause physical and mental problems connected with stress. Many disorders have a physical origin: they are linked to stress hormones generated in reaction to events that the brain has recognised as threatening. As we will see in the following chapters, our brain plays an important function in assisting us in surviving: it

4

assists us in detecting hazards in our surroundings. When the brain recognises a potentially dangerous scenario, it initiates a series of events that culminate in creating stress hormones. These hormones allow us to perform one of two things in the face of danger: fight or flee.

Both of these processes need the expenditure of energy. The two stress hormones provide us with the energy to combat the threat or leave if the risk is too high. Because of this great response, we were able to hunt mammoths in prehistoric times or flee successfully when they were too large.

However, research has revealed that when these hormones are released, they can return to the brain and influence our memory and emotional regulation by acting on brain areas involved in these tasks. Because of the effects of stress hormones on the body and the brain, the continued and large production of these hormones is at the root of various physical and mental problems linked with chronic stress.

And here is the essential knowledge that has come out of the last century's scientific research of stress. Researchers discovered that a scenario must include at least one of four criteria to elicit a stress response that might have long-term negative consequences. With any of these four traits, it makes no difference who you are—whatever your gender, age, or job, you will generate stress hormones every time.

The researchers also proved that a circumstance does not have to include all four features to elicit a stress response, but the release of stress hormones rises the more of these factors are there.

2

Why Does Living A Simple Life
Make People Happier?

EVERYONE DESIRES a happy and satisfying life. However, it appears that most of us seek pleasure in the wrong areas - money, celebrity, possessions, and decadence. We eventually find ourselves anxious, dissatisfied, and unhappy.

Why? Because we like to complicate things and overlook the fact that happiness is inextricably linked with simplicity. However, when we allow ourselves to think and ask ourselves what matters to us, we discover that a simple existence is preferable. And we begin to recognise what is essential to us. There are no huge milestones, large amounts of material, money, or luxury items required to experience pleasure. Finding beauty in life's modest pleasures and recognising that simplicity is the core of enjoyment is what life is all about. So, instead of seeking more things and managing hectic schedules, why not focus on what you have? Why not start enjoying life instead of just making a livelihood? After all, you deserved it!

Contrary to what marketers would have us think, acquiring more possessions, everlasting youth, additional wealth, or drinking a specific beer brand does not make people happy. According to extensive study in the emerging subject of positive psychology, real happiness (the sort that doesn't fade or alter with circumstances) comes from within ourselves in the form of self-esteem, social connections, humour, free time, and giving ourselves in service work or volunteering. These "drivers of happiness" are natural traits inside our psyches that may be cultivated to generate real effects, not just of increased happiness but also of increased productivity, life-span, health, and personal fulfilment in astonishingly short periods. Happiness does not come from adding more possessions or events to our lives; rather, it is the result of our mindset; the meaning we assign to events, what we choose to focus on, what beliefs we choose to embrace, and how we respond to daily challenges all play impor-tant roles in determining our baseline level of happiness. Everything we need to improve our happiness is here in front of us; there is no need to "obtain" anything else to be happy right now.

The science of happiness is now providing us with volumes of outstanding empirical data that supports the perspective of the ages' mystics, sages, and saints - that happiness comes first, and having the mindset and experiences of happiness is what creates the condi-tions that will attract the external "things" we want and believe will make us happy. It doesn't work the other way around.

Most of us have a habit of postponing our happiness, believing that when we have the ideal partner, money, body, and so on, we will be happy... at the same time; we wrongly believe that pleasure is a luxury item rather than a necessity. For example, when faced with time restrictions at work or school, one of our initial instincts is to abandon time spent with family and friends and hunker down in solitude to get the task done - a behaviour that appears to increase available time and attention to focus on the problem at hand. In reality, this reaction leads to emotions of being alone, isolated, and powerless; we become sad and stressed out, and since we've sepa-rated ourselves from one of our most significant happiness boosters, our social support network, our problem-solving talents are substan-tially diminished. Not the joyful ending we were hoping for!

Consider ourselves to be generals about to go into war or sportsmen about to compete in a huge game: to perform well; we must psychologically prepare ourselves for the obstacles ahead. In the pages that follow, we'll uncover our happy secret: a minimalist mentality.

This section is all about attitude. Before we can take control of our belongings, we must first modify our connection with them. We'll define it, explore what it is and isn't, and look at how it affects our lives. The concepts we learn will simplify us to let go of things and prevent more from entering the house. Most importantly, we will see that our possessions exist to serve us, not the other way around.

See Your Stuff For What It Is

Take a glance about you; there are probably at least twenty or thirty items in your direct line of sight. What exactly is this stuff? How did it get there? What is its function?

It's time to see our items for what they truly are. We want to identify it, define it, and remove the mystery around it. What are these things that we spend so much time and effort obtaining, managing, and storing? And how did there come to be so many? (Did they multiply while we were sleeping?)

In general, our belongings may be classified into three categories: useful stuff, beautiful stuff, and emotional stuff.

Let's start with the most basic category: useful items. These are the objects that are useful, functional and assist us in getting things done. Some are necessary for survival, while others make our lives a bit simpler. It's tempting to believe that everything we own is useful —but have you ever read a book on survival techniques? (If this is all you have, stop reading now; if not, join the rest of us and keep reading!) it's incredible how little we need to survive: a modest shelter, clothes to regulate our body temperature, food, water, a few containers, and some cooking tools.

Beyond the absolute necessities, some goods aren't strictly necessary for survival but are nonetheless extremely useful: beds, sheets, computers, tea kettles, combs, pencils, staplers, lights, books, plates, forks, sofas, extension cables, hammers, screwdrivers, whisks—you get the idea. Anything you use frequently and that brings value to your life is welcome in a minimalist household.

But keep in mind that to be useful, a thing must be utilised. That's the catch: most of us have many potentially beneficial items that we just do not utilise. Duplicates are an excellent example: how many of those plastic food containers make it from your cupboard to your lunch bag or freezer? Is your cordless drill actually in need of a backup? Food processors, fondue sets, and humidifiers are examples of items that languish because they are too complex or difficult to clean. Then there are the "just in case" and "may need it" items that lurk in the backs of our drawers, ready to make their appearance. Those are the things whose lives are counted.

Intermixed among our useful items are some that serve no practical use but satisfy a different type of need: to put it simply, we enjoy looking at them. We humans have always felt driven to enhance our environment, as shown by Palaeolithic cave drawings and the paintings that hang over our sofas.

Aesthetic enjoyment is a vital aspect of our identities that should not be overlooked. The dazzling glaze on a lovely vase or the sleek lines of a modernist chair may provide us profound and happy delight; hence, such objects have every right to be a part of our life. The caveat is that they must be revered and appreciated by being given a prominent position in our houses. If your Murano glass collection is gathering dust on a shelf or, worse, is kept in the attic, it is nothing more than colourful clutter.

Don't give anything artsy a free pass when you're going through your belongings. Just because something attracted you at a craft fair one summer day doesn't imply it merits a permanent lease on your living room mantel. If, on the other hand, it always brings a smile to your face—or if its visual harmony stirs your spirit with a greater appreciation for the beauty of life—it deserves a place in your house.

So, where did they come from, and what are they doing there? This would be simple if everything in our homes were either beautiful or helpful. But, as sure as the day is long, there will be plenty of goods that are neither. They symbolise some memory or emotional attachment nine times out of ten: your grandmother's old china, your father's pipe collection, the sarong you got on your honeymoon. They remind us of people, places, and events that have special meaning for us. They frequently enter our homes as presents, antiques, and souvenirs.

Again, if the thing in question brings you delight, show it

proudly and appreciate its presence. If, on the other hand, you're keeping it out of obligation (like Aunt Edna would turn over in her grave if you gave away her porcelain teacups) or proof of an experience (like nobody would believe you visited the Grand Canyon if you got rid of the kitschy snow globe), then some soul-searching is in order.

Talk to your belongings as you stroll about your house. "Who are you, and what do you do?" ask each item. "How did you enter my life?" "Did I purchase you, or were you given to me?" "How frequently do I use you?" "Would I replace you if you were lost or broken, or would I be pleased to have you gone?" "Did I ever want you in the first place?" You won't hurt your stuff's feelings if you're honest with your responses.

You'll most likely come across two sub-categories of things when asking these questions, one of which is "other stuff's stuff." You know what I mean: certain things just organically gather more stuff, such as accessories, manuals, cleaners, and items that go with the stuff, show the stuff, contain the junk, and fix the stuff. There's a lot of decluttering potential here: getting rid of one item might result in a cascade of leftovers!

"Other people's stuff" is the second sub-category. This is a difficult one. With the probable exception of your (young) children, you have very little power over other people's property. If it's the kayak your brother requested you to store in your basement and hasn't retrieved in fifteen years, you have the right to intervene (after a phone call requesting prompt removal, of course). When it comes to your spouse's excessive hobby supplies or your teen's outgrown pop star memorabilia, though, a more diplomatic approach is necessary. Hopefully, your decluttering will spread and result in those other individuals taking care of their belongings.

For now, simply go around and get to know your surroundings: that item is helpful, that one is lovely, and that one belongs to someone else (simple as pie!). Don't worry about decluttering just yet; we'll get to that later. Of course, if you manage to come across anything worthless, unattractive, or unidentifiable, go ahead and give it the boot!

In contrast to what some marketers would have you think, you are not your possessions. You are you, and things are things; no physical or mathematical alchemy can change these bounds, no matter what that full-page magazine ad or smart commercial claims.

Nonetheless, we are occasionally taken in by the advertiser's pitch. As a result, we must account for another type of object we own: "aspirational goods." These are the items we purchase to impress others or satisfy our "dream selves"—you know, the ones that are twenty pounds lighter, travel the world, attend cocktail parties, or perform in a rock band.

We may be uncertain to acknowledge it, but many of our belongings were most certainly purchased to portray a specific image. Take, for example, cars. We can meet our transportation needs with a basic automobile from point A to point B. So why would we spend twice (or even three times) the price for a "luxury" car? Because automakers invest large sums of money in advertising agencies to persuade us that our vehicles reflect ourselves, our personalities, and our places in the business world or social hierarchy.

Of course, it doesn't end there. The need to identify with commercial items pervades every aspect of our lives, from where we live to what we put in them. Most individuals would agree that a modest, simple dwelling meets our need for shelter more than adequately (especially compared to Third World accommodations). Aspirational marketing, on the other hand, dictates that we "need" a master suite, bedrooms for each child, his-and-her baths, and kitchens with professional-grade appliances; otherwise, we haven't quite "made it." Square footage becomes a prestige symbol, and consequently, a larger house needs many more sofas, chairs, tables, knickknacks, and other items.

We are told that the contents of our houses are reflections of ourselves and that we should take care to showcase the "correct" items to create the appropriate image. Bear rugs and deer antler chandeliers reflect our outdoorsy, pioneer attitude; Old World antiques reflect our sophisticated European preferences; Moroccan lanterns and floor pillows reflect our exotic, bohemian side. However, none of these items is required to express our interests or personalities; what we do, rather than what we have, is considerably more enlightening.

Advertisements also urge us to distinguish ourselves via our clothing, with brand name clothing. These expensive labels do not make our clothing warmer, our bags more durable, or our lives more glamorous. Furthermore, such trend-setting products appear to fall out of style mere minutes after purchase, leaving our wardrobes stuffed with out-of-date duds that we hope may return to vogue someday. Most of us don't need celebrity-sized wardrobes because our clothing and accessories will never be seen or commented on. Nonetheless, marketers attempt to persuade us that we live in the spotlight and should dress accordingly.

Being a minimalist in a media-saturated society is difficult. Advertisers continually bombard us with the notion that material possessions are the ultimate measure of success. They take advantage of the reality that it is far simpler to purchase status than acquire it. How many times have you heard the expressions "more is better," "fake it 'til you make it," or "clothes make the man?" They tell us that more stuff equals more happiness, but in reality, more stuff equals more headaches and debt. Someone will undoubtedly benefit from the acquisition of all of these things... But it isn't us.

Items can never transform us into someone we are not. Designer handbags will not make us wealthy, premium lipstick will not make us supermodels, and pricey pens will not make us effective executives. Pricey gardening equipment will not make us into green thumbs, and expensive cameras will not convert us into award-winning photographers. Nonetheless, we feel tempted to acquire and maintain things that claim to make us happier, prettier, smarter, a better parent or husband, more loved, more organised, or more capable.

But consider this: if these things haven't yet delivered on their promises, it's time to let them go.

Similarly, consumer goods are not stand-ins for the experience.

We don't need a garage full of camping equipment, sports equipment, and pool toys when all we truly want is quality time with our families. Inflatable reindeer and heaps of presents do not make for a happy holiday; but, meeting with our loved ones does. Accumulating mountains of yarn, piles of cookbooks, and bins of art supplies will not turn us become expert knitters, master cooks, or creative geniuses. The activities themselves, rather than the resources, are critical to our happiness and personal growth.

We often identify with items from our history and keep them to prove who we were or what we accomplished. How many of us still have cheerleading uniforms, letter sweaters, swimming medals, or notes from lengthy college classes? We justify preserving them as proof of our accomplishments (as if we might need to dig out our old Calculus tests to prove we passed the course). These artefacts, however, are generally stuffed in a box somewhere, without proving anything to anyone. If that's the case, it might be time to let go of these relics of your former self.

When we examine our possessions with a critical eye, we may be astonished at how much it remembers our history, symbolises our future dreams or belongs to our imaginary self. Unfortunately, spending too much of our attention, energy, and space on these things prevents us from living in the moment.

We sometimes worry that getting rid of particular objects is the same as getting rid of a piece of ourselves. No matter how infrequently we play the violin or wear that evening gown—the moment we let them go, we forfeit our potential to become virtuosos or socialites. And if we throw away our high school diploma, it will be as if we never graduated.

We must remember that our memories, dreams, and goals are not housed in these items; rather, they are stored within ourselves. We are not our possessions; we are what we do, think, and love. We make place for new (and actual) possibilities by removing the remnants of unloved pastimes, unfinished efforts, and unmet aspirations. Aspirational goods are the props for a fictional version of our life; we must clean out this clutter to have the time, energy, and space to actualise our genuine selves and full potential.

Less Stuff Equals Less Stress

Consider how much energy is expended in owning a single possession: preparing for it, reading reviews about it, seeking for the greatest price on it, earning (or borrowing) the money to purchase it, travelling to the store to buy it, carrying it home, finding a space for it, learning how to utilise it, cleaning it (or cleaning around it), maintaining it, buying extra parts for it, ensuring it, protecting it. Multiply this figure by the number of objects in your home. Whoa! That must be exhausting!

Being the keeper of all our possessions may be a full-time job. Entire companies have sprung up to assist us in servicing our possessions. Companies earn a fortune offering us specialist cleaning chemicals for every item—detergents for our clothing, silver polishes, furniture waxes, spray dusters for our gadgets, and leather conditioners. The insurance industry thrives on the possibility that our vehicles, jewels, or art will be damaged or stolen. Locksmiths, alarm providers, and safe manufacturers all claim to keep our belongings secure from robbery. When our stuff breaks, repairmen are standing by to fix it, and movers are ready to gather it up and transport it somewhere else.

With all of the time, money, and energy it necessitates, we may begin to believe that our possessions own us rather than the other way around. Let's take a deeper look at how much of our stress may be related to material possessions. First and foremost, we are concerned with a lack of material possessions. Maybe we saw something at a store or in an advertisement, and suddenly we can't picture our lives without it. Our neighbour has one, our sister received one as a present, and our coworker just bought one last week; are we the only ones who don't have one in the world? A sensation of deprivation begins to set in...

So now we're worried about how to get this item. Unfortunately, we don't know anyone who will give us one, so we'll have to get one for ourselves. We travel from store to store (or browse from website to website) to compare prices, hoping for a sale. We know we can't afford it right now, but we want it immediately. So we save some money, work additional hours, or charge it to a credit card, hoping to make the payments later.

The joyful day arrives when we finally purchase it. At long last, it is ours! The sun is shining, birds are chirping, and all of your worries have vanished. Right? Consider it again. We'll have to take good care of it now that we've spent a lot of money on it. We've taken on not just a new possession but also a new level of duty.

We must keep it clean regularly since dust and grime might impair its performance and shorten its lifespan. We must keep it out of reach of children and dogs. We must use extreme caution when using it to avoid breaking, ruining, or staining it. Sound crazy? How many times did you park a new car at the far end of a car park or had your day spoiled by a dent or scratch? How did you feel after splattering tomato sauce over your costly silk blouse?

Then, when anything goes wrong with it, which is unavoidable, we worry about fixing it. We read over instruction manuals or search the Internet for answers. We go out and purchase the necessary tools or new parts for the repair. We drag it into a repair shop when we fail. Or perhaps we postpone because we don't know how (or don't want to) deal with it. It lurks in a corner, a closet, or the basement, weighing on our minds. Perhaps we didn't break it but just grew tired of it. In any case, we're feeling a little guilty and anxious about spending so much time and money on it.

Then we watch another advertisement and are attracted by something completely different; this one is even more intriguing than the previous one. Oh-oh, here we go again...

We never seem to have enough time in our days—perhaps it's because of our possessions. How many hours have we squandered rushing to the dry cleaners, how many Saturdays have we given up for oil changes or car repairs, how many days off have we spent mending or maintaining our belongings (or waiting for a specialist to make a service call)? How often have we worried (or reprimanded our children) over a shattered vase, a chipped plate, or mud stains on our area rugs? How much time have we wasted looking for cleaners, replacement parts, and accessories for the items we currently own?

Let's take a moment to reflect on how carefree and joyful we were in college. Not by chance, that was also the time when we had the least amount of goods. There was no mortgage, no vehicle payments, and no motorboat to insure back then. Learning, living, and having fun were far more essential than material possessions. Everything was conceivable since the world was our oyster! That is the delight we can reclaim as minimalists. We simply need to put our things in its proper location so that it does not take up the majority of our attention.

That doesn't mean we have to live in studio flats furnished with milk crates and used couches. Instead, for the time being, suppose that we only had half of what we have today. That is a big relief in and of itself! That equates to 50% less effort and anxiety! 50% less cleaning, maintenance, and repair! Credit card debt has been reduced by 50%! What will we do with all of this additional time and money? Ah, the light bulb has gone off... We're starting to notice the benefits of becoming minimalists.

Less Stuff Equals Greater Freedom

What if you were offered a fantastic, once-in-a-lifetime opportunity —but you had to relocate across the nation in three days to accept it? Would you be ecstatic and begin making plans? Or would you glance about your house, concerned about how you were going to have everything packed up in time? Would you be horrified by the prospect of transferring your belongings hundreds of miles (or, worse, think it ridiculous)? How probable is it that you'll conclude it's not worth the trouble, that you've "settled" here, and that some-thing else will come along some other time?

It may sound absurd to think, but might your possessions have the ability to keep you in place? For many of us, the answer is likely to be "yes."

Things may act as anchors. They can bind us and prevent us from pursuing new interests and developing new abilities. They can interfere with relationships, job advancement, and family time. They have the potential to sap our vitality and feeling of adventure.

16

Have you ever avoided a social gathering because your home was too messy for the company? Have you ever missed a child's rugby game because you were working extra hours to make credit card payments? Have you ever been rejected on an exotic trip because there was no one to "keep an eye on the house?"

Examine everything in the room where you're seated. Consider each of these objects—each possession—to be connected to you with a piece of rope. Some are attached to your arms, some to your waist, and yet more to your legs. (For added drama, imagine shackles instead.) Try getting up and moving about with all of this junk dragging, clinging, and clanging behind you. Not so simple, is it? You won't be able to go very far or do very much. It won't be long until you give up, sit down, and realise it's far easier to stay where you are.

Similarly, too much clutter may dampen our emotions. It's as if each of those objects has its gravitational field that always pushes us down and keeps us back. We might physically feel heavy and sluggish in a crowded environment, too tired and lazy to get up and do anything. In contrast, a clean, bright, minimally decorated room makes us feel light, emancipated, and full of possibilities.

We feel energised and ready for anything now that all of our possessions do not burden us.

With this in mind, we may be tempted to implement a fast fix to create the appearance of a clean space. We'll just go down to the superstore, get some nice containers, and create a minimalist space right now. Unfortunately, putting everything into drawers, baskets, and bins will not suffice: out of sight, out of mind does not apply here. Even things that are hidden away (whether in a hall closet, the basement, or across town in a storage facility) remain in the back of our minds. We must completely shake off things to be psychologically free.

Another thing to consider: in addition to physically crowding and psychologically suffocating us, possessions also financially imprison us through the debt we incur to pay for them. The more money we owe, the more restless nights we have and the fewer possibilities we have. Getting up every morning and dragging ourselves to jobs we don't enjoy to pay for things we may no longer have, utilise, or even desire isn't easy. There are so many other things we'd rather be doing! Furthermore, if we've spent our salaries (and then some) on consumer goods, we've depleted our resources for other rewarding activities, such as taking an art class or investing in a new business.

Travel is an excellent parallel for the liberation of a minimalist life. Consider how inconvenient it is to lug about two or three big suitcases when on vacation. You've been looking forward to this vacation for a long time, and as you get off the aircraft, you can't wait to explore the sites. Not so fast—you must first wait (and wait) for your luggage to emerge on the luggage carousel. Then it would help if you transported them through the airport. You might as well take a taxi because navigating them on the metro would be virtually impossible. And forget about getting a head start on sightseeing— you must go straight to your hotel to relieve yourself of this enormous burden. You fall in exhaustion when you finally reach there.

Minimalism, on the other hand, improves your agility. Consider travelling with little more than a light backpack—the experience is wonderfully thrilling. You rush from the plane and zip through the crowds waiting for your bags when you arrive at your location. Then you may take the metro, a bus or begin walking in the direction of your hotel. Along the journey, you get to see, hear and smell the sights, sounds, and fragrances of a new city, and you have the time and energy to appreciate it all. You're as mobile, adaptable, and free as a bird, able to carry your luggage to museums and tourist attractions and stash it in a locker when necessary.

In contrast to the previous scenario, you struck the ground running and spent the afternoon sightseeing rather than dragging your belongings. You return to your hotel invigorated by your adventure and eager for more.

It's the same with life. When we surround ourselves with stuff, we become like tourists in a cab, shut off from other people and all the exciting things around us. Our belongings pile up to form a cage around us. We reclaim our freedom by dismantling these dungeons piece by item as we become minimalists. We can appreciate life, connect with people, and engage in our communities when our possessions no longer bind us. We're more open to new experiences and better equipped to spot and capitalise on possibilities. The less baggage we carry (both physically and mentally), the more we can live!

How Do I Start Living A Simple Life?

ONE OF THE best parts about making your life simpler is that it doesn't have to be expensive or time-consuming. You can reduce the complexity in your life one step at a time and yet obtain fantastic outcomes. As with any successful activity, certain broad, tried-and-true rules are useful to understand and follow. These ideas apply whether you're at home, at work, or in Timbuktu. But it is at home you have the most power, the most belongings, and the opportunity to put these ideas into action late at night or on weekends.

While the ideas in this chapter and the recommendations throughout the book can assist you, you must grasp the following: There is no absolute unified theory of simplicity, just as Albert Einstein was unable to develop a unified explanation of the world. What is straightforward for one individual may be difficult and time-consuming for you. So, assess any simple advice you come across in terms of what will work for you.

There Will Be No Spontaneous Piles

A fundamental step in making your life easier is to face the heaps in your life with a no-holds-barred approach. Some heaps will accumulate in every life. These piles contain stacks of periodicals, newspapers, bills, reports, paperwork, certifications, school notices, homework, photos, and other items. If you haven't observed, such heaps may quickly build. A couple of issues of a magazine, some coupons clipped from the newspaper, a single day's worth of mail, some fliers left by your door, the electric bill from a few days ago, and you've got yourself a pile.

By definition, a pile represents complexity. The more complicated the pile symbolises, the taller the stack and the more diversified the parts that comprise it. Don't be shocked if some researcher discovers a relationship between the number of piles one collects and the prevalence of heart disease. Piles indicate unfinished business and, as a result, a failure to complete one's affairs. Each pile you come across registers in your brain, if only for a nanosecond, as additional things you haven't dealt with.

Get Out From Under Those Piles Using A Shovel

According to organisational experts, an accumulation of items indicates a lack of decision-making. Simply adding anything to a jumble of other things takes up space and limits your psychological mobility. Fortunately, there are several approaches to dealing with the ad hoc piles that appear all too regularly in your life.

Get a full night's sleep before launching your assault; if your piles resemble the Grand Tetons—you'll need the energy. Then proceed with the procedures below to drive the piles into the earth.

1. Gather a pen, a few file folders, some paper clips, rubber bands, and a stapler. Now, take those problematic piles (using a wheelbarrow if required) and transport them to a work location such as your kitchen table or a desk. Stack them all in front of you in a temporary pile. Check your watch and give yourself 30 minutes or less to deconstruct and reallocate this simplicity-threatening mountain into four smaller stacks: one for important items, one for urgent items, one for interesting items, and one for the recycling bin (where most items will go).

2. Don't spend too much time worrying about which pile to put each thing in. Allocate to the best of your ability. Place an item towards the top of the important pile if it is urgent and vital. Place

it in the urgent pile if it is simply urgent. If you're not sure about an item, put it near the bottom of the original big stack. Do not repeat this process for each item. Make a decision the next time you go through the initial stack. The substantial mound should be gone in 30 minutes or less, leaving you with four semi-neat small piles. Get rid of the recycling pile.

Finally, you'll have three tiny, neatly organised piles of vital, urgent, and fascinating material. Then, arrange the things in ascending order in the remaining piles, with the most important at the top. Downgrade or toss anything you can. You're probably already feeling better.

3. As you examine and reorganise the three task piles you've constructed, keep in mind that you can always get meaner, leaner, and more concentrated. What else can you chuck? What may be merged, disregarded, postponed, delegated, rented out, mechanised, systemised, or used as kindling? The more stuff you can downgrade to intriguing, the further ahead you will be since you will be able to deal with these objects anytime you choose.

4. Once you've reduced the number of your piles and arranged them into slender, trim form, store-like items together. Staplers, paper clips, rubber bands, and other organisational tools can be used. In general, the more similar objects you can tie together, the easier it will be to discover any specific item you want.

5. Begin with the most critical pile and estimate how long each item will take to complete. Add together all of your estimations and multiply the total by 1.5. (This allows for the majority of people's habitual underestimate.) Repeat with the remaining piles. As the task hours mount up, you'll realise how serious the pile-building behaviour is. Your new approach to the job at hand will differ depending on what you want to accomplish, the assistance available, and other factors unique to your situation.

Become A Task Master

Once you've reduced the mounds that plagued your home to a few meticulously sorted stacks, you're ready to tackle the jobs that survived the weeding-out process. Here are some suggestions to help you get there. Take each item one at a time. Begin working on the essential project or job (the one at the top of the important folder) after you've selected it. If you are unable to complete it—perhaps with the assistance of others—continue with it as far as you are able. Then return it to the stack, either on top or wherever you believe it currently belongs. Similarly, start with the next most crucial thing and work your way up.

Change it up. When you need a break from working on critical tasks, switch to the urgent stack. Examine the intriguing pile relatively seldom, possibly once every couple of days or weeks. It's fine if the intriguing pile becomes thick. You'll eventually categorise or discard its contents.

Reduce the volume. A little mound of stuff is easier to manage than a massive pile. Always attempt to preserve just the information that you feel is necessary. Make every effort to decrease the size, weight, and volume of each pile. Instead of maintaining a five-page report, keep only the one page that you truly need. Rather than keeping the full page, cut the paragraph, address, phone number, or essential information you require and discard the rest. Tape the little clipping you've saved to a page with additional pertinent information.

Allow piles to accumulate in rare instances. When is it alright to let certain piles expand, mirror, mirror on the wall? When they represent similar objects, the response is yes. For example, maybe everything in a stack is linked to your child's schooling, or the pile is transitory, and you fully intend to organise it within a specific time frame. Even under these conditions, a pile can be reduced. Go on a mission of search and destroy. Look for duplicate information and discard it.

Everything should be reexamined in a new light. Even after you've reduced a pile to a smaller, more concise pile, go through it again with this question in mind: What am I still holding on to that adds unnecessary complexity? Perhaps you are already aware of the issue represented by an item and do not need to save printed information about it. From that vantage, you might be able to toss a third or more of the documents left in your already-stripped-down pile.

Make a list of keywords. Simple words and phrases that are

written on a single piece of paper can replace pages and pages of stuff. If you have items in your pile that just act as reminders to you, then a list of key terms might be more useful. This chapter's key terms, for example, contained "ad hoc piles," "unfinished business," "information crutches," "keywords," "holding bins," and "giveaway boxes," among others.

Arrange your piles such that they are easily accessible. If you've reduced the number of piles, consider arranging them in a cascading or stair-step pattern down one side of your desk or table. The top inch of each would be visible before being covered by the next. This configuration allows you to draw from any of the piles while maintaining the others in order.

Get them out of the way. Many people claim that storing their stacks of documents will cause them to lose track of them. You don't have to spread out your stacks to find them. Use file cabinets, desk drawers, and other storage options to keep items out of sight yet conveniently accessible. Only use a visible layout of your piles on a desktop if you deal with the piles quickly.

Detach Yourself From Your Possessions

The great haiku poet Basho stated,

"Since my house burned down,
   I now have a clearer view.
   Of the rising moon."

That's someone who isn't attached to his possessions!

While we don't have to go to such lengths, we might benefit from cultivating a comparable feeling of non-attachment. Developing such an attitude would make it much simpler to declutter our houses and lessen the sorrow when items are removed from us through other ways (such as theft, flood, fire, or a collection agency).

We'll need to stretch, limber up, and get in shape for the job ahead if we want to meet our objectives. As a result, we'll spend this chapter practising mental exercises to relax our grasp on our belongings. We'll strengthen our minimalist muscles in the following pages while also developing the psychological power and flexibility required for a battle with our belongings.

To get ourselves fired up, let's envision life without our possessions. This is simple—we don't even need to imagine it; we can remember it.

Many of us remember our adolescence as one of the happiest, most carefree periods of our life. Even though we lived in a shoebox (often with two or three other people) with minimal disposable income, however, we couldn't afford fashionable clothes, expensive watches, or technological gadgets. Everything we had fit into a few boxes, and we didn't have to worry about car repairs, home maintenance, or even going to the dry cleaners. Our social life took precedence over whatever little we possessed. We were carefree and fancy-free!

Do you believe such liberty is a thing of the past? No, not always. Many of us get the opportunity to revisit our "stuff-free" lifestyles once or twice a year when we go on vacation. In reality, the word vacation is derived from the Latin 'vacare', which means "to be empty." It's no surprise that we want to get away from it all!

Consider the last time you went camping, for example. In your pack, you carried everything you needed for both comfort and survival. You were unconcerned about your looks and got by just fine with the clothes on your back. You ate with little more than a plate, cup, and fork and cooked your meal in a portable pan over an open fire. Your tent, the most basic kind of shelter, kept you warm and dry. Your few belongings matched your requirements, giving you plenty of time to rest and communicate with nature.

So why do we require so much more when we return to our "actual" lives? We don't—and that's the idea of these activities. We'll realise that much of what surrounds us isn't required for our health and pleasure.

Now that you've warmed up let's take things to the next level and imagine you're going abroad. But don't call your local self-storage facility just yet—this is a permanent move. You can't merely put your belongings away in preparation for your return. Furthermore, shipping things worldwide is complicated and expensive, so you'll have to limit yourself to what you must have.

Examine the contents of your home and determine what you'll take. Would your beat-up old guitar cut? How about your collection of ceramic animals? Would you give up valuable cargo space for an unattractive sweater you got three Christmases ago, shoes that hurt your feet after fifteen minutes, or an oil painting you inherited but never liked? Certainly not! Isn't it wonderful? It's surprising what you can get rid of when you suddenly have "permission!"

Okay, you're on your game now, so let's try a difficult one: it's the middle of the night, and you're jolted awake by the piercing sound of the fire alarm. Oh my goodness! You just have a few minutes, if not seconds, before you leave the house to determine what you'll save. To be sure, you'll have few options here and will have to depend primarily on instinct. You may take some essential documents, a family photo book, and possibly your laptop if you have the time. In all likelihood, you'll have to give up everything to save yourself, your family, and your pets. At that moment, you won't give a whit about all the things that have previously absorbed your attention.

Whew! Let's take a breather after that one to allow our heartbeats to settle down. We're going to slow them down a lot... till they stop. What!

As much as we hate to think about it, our time on Earth will come to an end at some point, and sadly, it may come sooner than we expect. And what will happen after that? People are going to go through our belongings. Yikes! It's a good thing we won't be able to blush since that would be humiliating. Whether we like it or not, the items we leave behind become part of our legacy, and I doubt any of us want to be remembered as junk collectors or packrats. Wouldn't you rather be known for living simply and elegantly, with only the essentials and a few treasured items?

Take some time to mentally inventory your "estate." What story do your belongings say about you? Hopefully, it isn't anything like, "Boy, she had a thing for takeaway cartons" or "That's weird, I didn't realise he collected old calendars." Do your heirs a favour, and don't let them sift through a cluttered residence after your demise. Otherwise, when you look down from the hereafter, you'll probably find folks rummaging through your "treasures" at a massive yard sale.

Okay, I swear there will be no more sadness and gloom—this is a cheerful book! The idea is that a break from our daily routines (whether from a vacation or a natural disaster) helps us put our problems into perspective, and in the latter instance, it's far better to envision it than to really experience it. Such scenarios let us understand that our stuff isn't all that essential in the great scheme of things, and with that awareness, we may decrease its hold on us and be ready (and willing) to let it go.

Be An Effective Gatekeeper

One of my favourite minimalist quotations is by British writer and designer William Morris, who said, *Have nothing in your houses that you do not know to be necessary or consider to be beautiful.* It's a lovely sentiment, but how can we put it into action? After all, we don't bring unnecessary or unattractive objects into our houses on purpose; still, certain less-than-desirable manage to make their way in. The solution is for us to become better gatekeepers.

It's not that difficult. Things enter our homes in one of two ways: we purchase them or are given to us (in other words, we get them for free). They don't come in while we're not looking, no matter how much we'd want to believe. They don't appear out of nowhere, nor do they reproduce behind our backs (except perhaps the paperclips and Tupperware). Unfortunately, the blame falls completely on our shoulders: we allowed them in.

As you go through your belongings, consider how each thing came into your life. Did you go out of your way to find it, pay for it, and eagerly carry it back to your house or apartment? Did it follow you home from that Birmingham conference or that trip to Benidorm? Or did it creep in under the cover of colourful paper and a beautiful bow?

Our homes are our castles, and we spend a lot of money defending them. We apply pesticides to keep pests out, use air filters to keep pollutants out and have security systems to keep intruders out. What are we overlooking? A clutter blocker to keep the clutter at bay! We must take matters into our own hands since I have yet to see such a product on the market (and if one does come in the future, you heard it here first).

Of course, we have total control over what we acquire; all we have to do is use it. Don't lower your guard when anything falls into your cart. Don't bring anything to the checkout line without thoroughly investigating it. Ask yourself (in your head!) the following questions about each possible purchase: "Are you worthy of a place in my home?" "How will you offer value to my household?" "Are you willing to make my life easier?" "Or will you be more bother than you're worth?" "Do I have a spot for you?" "Do I already have anything that could do the same function?" "Will I want to retain you forever (or at least for an extended period)?" "How difficult will it be to get rid of you if not?" The final question alone spared me from carrying a bag full of souvenirs from China home—because once anything has memories, it's a pain to get rid of.

That's not that tough, is it? All we have to do is pause and ask ourselves, "Why?" before we buy. But what about the things we don't choose to obtain and, in many cases, don't even want? (I'm looking at you, gifts, freebies, and promotional stuff!) It might be difficult (or impolite) to deny them; yet, once they have taken up residence in our houses, they can be much more difficult to expel.

When it comes to freebies, the best defence is a solid attack. Instead of magnets, pencils, and paperweights with company logos, take a business card. Turn down the perfume and cosmetic samples in the mall (hey, what are you doing at the mall?) and the supermarket's small detergents and dishwashing solutions. When opening a bank account, decline the toaster and request an equivalent cash deposit (it's certainly worth a try!). Learning to gently refuse them is a vital skill that comes in handy more frequently than you think.

If you're attending a professional meeting or conference, go over the booklets, pamphlets, and other materials while you're there; if they end up in your luggage, distribute them back at the office. And, please, leave the lotions, shampoos, and conditioners in the hotels where they belong. Don't allow these miniatures (as adorable as they are) to clutter up your cupboards and drawers unless you intend to utilise them.

Gifts, on the other hand, necessitate a different strategy. I've discovered that it's better to take things gracefully without going crazy with thanks (since if you make a big deal, you're bound to get something similar the following year). However, this creates a dilemma: what do you do with unwanted gifts? We don't want to stuff them into drawers or the backs of closets—after all, we're trying to declutter!

The remedy is straightforward:

- Never let them settle in.
- Keep a donation box outside of your living space (such as in the basement) and dispose of unneeded items there right away.
- When it's filled, take it to a local charity of your choice. The time delay between getting the item and giving it (while waiting for the box to fill up) might work to your advantage.

For example, if Aunt Margaret pays you a visit in the interim, you may immediately collect the bookends she gave you and place them on display. Photographing the present may also help: if it's a trinket, take a picture of it on your mantelpiece; if it's a sweater or scarf, put it on and pose for a picture. Send the photo to the gift giver and the item to charity, and joy will reign.

To be an effective gatekeeper, you must regard your home as a holy space rather than a storage space. You are not obligated to take in every stray thing that crosses your way. When one attempts to sneak or charm its way in, keep in mind that you have the authority to reject entry. If the thing isn't going to bring value to your life in terms of function or beauty, put up a "Sorry, No Vacancy" sign. A simple rejection now can save you hours of decluttering later!

Accept Space

For our purposes, we'll take a minimalist approach and declare, "Life is the space between our possessions." Too much clutter might hinder our creativity and disrupt our lives. In contrast, the more space we have, the more lovely and harmonious our lives may be. Space is nothing special, but we never seem to have enough of it. We are greatly distressed by the lack of it; in fact, we would do practically anything to have extra space in our homes, closets, and garages. We remember having more of it at some point in the past, and its absence is the reason for alarm. We look around, confused, and ask, "Where did all our space go?"

We have great recollections of how our homes appeared on the first day we moved in; wow, all that lovely space! But what transpired? It's not quite as stunning as we recall. Our space, on the other hand, did not vanish. It's still standing just where we left it. Our priorities changed, not the space. We were so preoccupied with other things that we entirely forgot about the space. We lost sight of the reality that the two are mutually exclusive: that a small amount of space is lost for every new object we bring into our houses. The issue is that we place a higher value on our possessions than on our living space.

The good news is that while space is easy to lose, it is also simple to regain. Get rid of something, and bingo! Space! Remove another thing, and there you have it! More room! This is great fun! Soon, all of those small places will add up to a large space, and we will be able to move about again. Make the most of your extra room by doing a joyful dance!

We must remember (and it is all too easy to forget) that the quantity of stuff we may possess is limited by the amount of space we have to store it. It's just basic physics. Nothing you stuff, squish, shove, or pull will change it. If you wish, you can seal everything up in "magic" vacuum bags, but even those have to go somewhere. So, if you live in a tiny apartment or don't have a lot of closet space, you can't carry many items home. Period. You'll have an issue if you don't.

We don't have to occupy every available area. Remember that space has the same value as objects (or greater, depending on your perspective). You don't need to accumulate four thousand square feet of things if you live in a four thousand square foot house. You don't have to stuff every inch of your walk-in closet if you have one. Really! If you don't, you'll be able to live and breathe a lot easier.

In the introduction, we discussed the importance of containers and how they have the most potential when they are empty. We need an empty cup to pour tea into when we wish to drink a cup of tea. We need an empty pot to cook a meal in when we wish to create one. When we want to dance the tango, we need an empty room.

Similarly, our homes serve as receptacles for our personal life. When we want to unwind, create, and play with our family, we need some open space to do so. Alternatively, we might consider our houses to be the stages on which our lives' dramas occur. We need to be able to move around and express ourselves freely to give our best performance; stumbling over props is never fun (or especially elegant).

We also require space for our ideas and thoughts—a messy home sometimes leads to a congested mind. Assume you're sitting on your sofa, possibly reading a book or listening to music, when a genuinely deep idea enters your mind: perhaps you've got an insight into human nature, or you're on the verge of discovering the meaning of life. When your eyes are drawn to the stack of magazines on the coffee table or the broken sewing machine in the corner, you are deep in thought, unravelling the riddles of mankind. "Hmm, I need to get to that," you think; "I wonder if there will be time before dinner..." Your mind quickly takes a detour, and your line of thought—and hence your legacy as a great philosopher—is lost.

Of course, you don't have to be Aristotle to appreciate a clean environment. Even routine occupations benefit immensely from space and clarity; for example, it is much simpler to devote your whole attention to your partner or kid when there aren't a million things around to confuse and distract you.

That is the best part about space: it highlights the things (and people) that are genuinely precious to us. If you had a great picture, you wouldn't overwhelm it with other decorations; instead, you'd display it alone, with enough space around it to show it off. If you possessed a beautiful vase, you wouldn't bury it under a mound of rubbish; instead, you'd place it on its pedestal. We need to treat what is essential to us with the same regard, which entails getting rid of anything else.

By making room in our houses, we emphasise where it belongs: what we do rather than what we own. Life is too short to waste it worrying over trivial matters. For when we're old and grey, we won't wax lyrical about the things we had—rather, we'll wax poetic about what we did in the gaps between them.

Have Fun Without Owning

What if someone offered you the Mona Lisa on the condition that you do not sell it? Sure, you'd have access to a magnificent picture 24 hours a day, but suddenly the responsibility for one of humanity's greatest assets would fall firmly on your shoulders. It would be a difficult effort to keep her safe from theft, clear of dust and dirt, sheltered from sunshine, and maintained at the ideal temperature and humidity. You'd also have to cope with a continuous stream of art enthusiasts who wanted to see her. Any joy you could receive from her possession would very certainly be overshadowed by the strain of her care and upkeep. That intriguing smile might not be so endearing for much longer.

On second thought, thanks but no thanks—we'll just leave her at the Louvre!

In our contemporary culture, we are extremely fortunate to have access to so many of humanity's masterpieces without buying and maintaining them ourselves. Our cities are such incredible art, culture, and entertainment providers that we don't need to recreate them within our own four walls.

One of the secrets to having a minimalist house is to explore new ways to "enjoy without owning." Consider the cappuccino makers gathering dust in our kitchen cabinets. In principle, being able to prepare a hot cup of frothy java in the comfort of our own homes is handy (and rather indulgent). The contraption is a hassle to pull out, set up, and clean up after we're done, and the brew never seems to taste as wonderful as it should. It's less special when we can get it whenever we want. After a few rounds of the barista, we realise it's more enjoyable to go to a local coffee shop and soak in the atmosphere while drinking our cup.

To live a minimalist lifestyle, we must fight the need to replicate the outside world within our homes. Unfortunately, house design trends have shifted in the opposite direction: media rooms, fitness centres, and bathroom "spas" are all the rage in the luxury home market. It's almost as if we're going to fortify ourselves and never leave our homes. Instead of buying, maintaining, and repairing all that equipment, why not reward yourself for a pleasant night out at the movies, a trip to the gym (or a stroll), or a day at the local spa? This way, you may enjoy such hobbies whenever they strike your fancy—without having to store and care for all of your belongings.

Apply the same technique to your backyard for even less labour and concern. Maintain it neatly, but don't feel forced to produce a botanical spectacular behind your house. Instead, do what city residents do and visit public parks and gardens. Professional landscapers perform all of the work there, leaving you free to enjoy the ever-changing landscape of flowers and greenery. It's a wonderful way to get your greens fix without owning a garage full of lawn and garden equipment. Similarly, there's no need to transform your backyard into a five-star resort with a pool, tennis courts, fire pit, and outdoor living rooms when you can get identical facilities (and much less care) at your local community centre or swim club.

If you're prone to purchase "beautiful" items, repeat "enjoy without owning" as a mantra when you're out shopping. Admire the delicate detail of a glass figurine, the metalwork on an antique bracelet, or the brilliant hues of an artisan vase—but instead of taking them home, leave them on display. Consider it similar to a museum visit: a chance to enjoy the beauty and design of well-crafted things without the prospect (or pressure) of ownership.

We aim to decrease the number of items in our houses that demand our care and attention as we strive to become minimalists. Fortunately, we have plenty of opportunities to do so by simply moving some of our joys and activities into the public domain. In reality, such activity has a fairly amazing secondary effect. We become substantially more socially active and civically involved when we spend time in parks, museums, movie theatres, and coffee shops rather than trying to recreate comparable experiences in our own homes. We can get out into the world and enjoy more direct,

direct, and fulfilling experiences by tearing down the material walls around us.

The Joy Of Enough

"He who realises he has enough is rich," stated Chinese philosopher Lao Tzu, author of the Tao Te Ching.

Enough—it's a slippery notion. What is sufficient for one person is insufficient for another, and what is sufficient for one person is excessive for another. Most of us would agree that we have enough food, drink, clothes, and shelter to satisfy our fundamental requirements. And everyone who reads this book is likely to believe that they have plenty. So, why do we still want to acquire and own more?

Let us look into the term "enough" a bit more closely. It is defined as "adequate for the want or need; sufficient for the purpose or to fulfil desire" by Dictionary.com. Ah, there's the rub: even after we've met our necessities, there's still the issue of our wants and wishes. That is where we must concentrate to feel the delight of "enough." It's pretty simple: pleasure is desiring what you have. When your wants are met by the items you already own, there is no need to purchase anything else. But desires may be annoying little creatures, and to regulate them, we must first understand what drives them.

Assume we live in the middle of nowhere, with no access to television or the Internet and no subscriptions to magazines or newspapers. We may live simply, but we are completely content with what we have. We're warm, well-fed, and out of physical danger. Simply put, we have enough. Then one day, a family constructs a house next door to us that is larger and more crowded than ours. Our no enough longer appears to be enough. Then more families move in, each with their own set of houses, cars, and belongings; holy cow, we had no idea how much stuff we didn't have! A satellite link provides access to TV and the Internet and a look into the opulent lifestyles of the affluent and famous. We still have the same belongings as before, with which we were perfectly content until now, but now we can't help but feel deprived.

What happened? We succumbed to the age-old issue of

"keeping up with the Joneses." Suddenly, we're not assessing "enough" in objective terms (is our house big enough for our family?) but in relative terms (is our house as lovely, huge, or new as the one next door?). Worse, the problem is exacerbated by the bar continuing rising; after we've reached the level of one Jones, we shift our attention to the next Jones up. But, let's face it: there will always be someone who has more than we do. So, unless we genuinely believe we will become the richest individuals in the world, defining our "wealth" in relation to others is a futile exercise. Even billionaires aren't immune to this tendency; they've been known to strive to outdo one other in terms of the size of their yachts. What's the point if happiness with things is out of grasp even at the highest levels?

The truth is that once we've met our fundamental requirements, the amount of stuff we own has very little to do with our pleasure. Beyond this point, the marginal value (or satisfaction) obtained from consuming further things decreases fast, and it even becomes negative at what economists term the "satiation point." (Perhaps that is why you are reading this book!) As a result, "more" frequently fail to please us—and, in certain circumstances, might even make us unhappy. As a result, consumer one-upmanship is a shell game in which the only winners are the firms selling the items. We'd be happier, more relaxed, and more fulfilled if we stopped doing it altogether.

Developing a grateful mindset is considerably more suited to a simple existence. We will not desire more if we realise the riches in our life and appreciate what we have. We simply need to concentrate on what we have rather than what we don't. If we are to draw comparisons, we must look globally and locally; we must look down and up the ladder. Even the poorest First World families are wealthy by Third World standards. So, while we may feel deprived compared to others in our own country who are richer, we live like royalty compared to many others worldwide.

Let's end off our topic of "enough" with a small exercise now that we have a better sense of where we are in the world (and not only in comparison to celebrities or our neighbours). It's extremely simple; all you'll need is paper and a pencil (or a computer, if you

35

prefer). Ready? Make a note of everything you possess and go around your house. I know some of you are looking at this page incredulously, but no, I'm not kidding. Make a list of everything in your house: every book, every plate, every fork, every garment, every shoe, every sheet, every pen, every knickknack—in short, everything. Is it too difficult? Try only one room. Still unable to complete the task? Let's say you just have one drawer. Isn't it a little overwhelming? Do you still get the feeling that you don't have enough?

Live Simply So Others May Live Simply

"Live simply, so that others may simply live," Mahatma Gandhi once wrote.

As it turns out, this may be the most compelling reason to become a minimalist.

Now that we're thinking on a larger scale consider this: we share this world with almost six billion other individuals. Our space and resources are limited. How do we ensure that there is enough food, water, land, and energy for everyone? By not utilising any more of it than we need. Because for every "extra" we take, someone else will have to do without (now or in the future). That "extra" may not make a major difference in our well-being, but it may be a matter of life and death for someone else.

We must recognise that we do not exist in a vacuum; the effects of our activities are felt all across the world. Would you still run the water while brushing your teeth if it meant that someone else would be thirsty? Would you continue to drive a gas-guzzling vehicle if you knew a global oil scarcity would result in poverty and chaos? Would you still build a large house if you saw the effects of deforestation firsthand? We might live a bit more lightly if we knew how our lives affect others.

Our purchasing habits have an impact on the environment. Every item we purchase, from food to books to televisions to automobiles, takes part of the earth's richness. Not only does its production and distribution necessitate the use of energy and natural resources, but its disposal is also a source of concern. Do we really want our grandkids to grow up amid massive landfills? The less we rely on to survive, the better off everyone (and our world) will be. As a result, we should cut back on our consumption as much as possible and prioritise items and packaging produced from minimum, biodegradable, or recyclable materials.

Our purchases also have a human cost. Unfortunately, global outsourcing has bred an out-of-sight, out-of-mind attitude toward this issue. Manufacturing has shifted away from our own towns, where we could witness firsthand the working conditions of our neighbours—and where we could rely on laws, unions, and other controls to safeguard and assure their safety. Things we buy are now manufactured on the other side of the world, where labour is cheap and few restrictions. When we buy anything, we should think about the people who produce it. What type of conditions did they work in? What impact did the manufacture of this item have on their lives, communities, and environment? Is our need (or desire) for this thing worth their pain if it is negative?

Of course, calculating the human and environmental effects of everything we purchase is nearly impossible. We should educate ourselves as best we can, but our study will never be exhaustive; manufacturers are rarely upfront about their foreign activities and frequently relocate to save money. It may take us months to acquire all of the necessary information for a single acquisition. We may, however, avoid this issue while still reducing our consumption foot-prints by shopping locally, buying used, and buying less.

Buying locally offers several ethical, environmental, and economic advantages:

Locally-made items are considerably more likely to have been created under fair and humane labour conditions.

Avoiding long-distance travel saves enormous amounts of energy. Buying vegetables from your local farmer's market, for example, is far better for the environment than having them shipped halfway around the world.

Supporting our local economy preserves our hard-earned funds in our communities, where they can be utilised to build infrastructure and provide services that improve our lives and the lives of our neighbours.

Buying secondhand allows us to get the items we need without placing further strain on the earth's resources. Why waste resources and energy on a new item when an old one would suffice? Rather than travelling to the mall, shop the used market for furniture, appliances, electronics, apparel, books, toys, and other items. Thrift stores, classified ads, and websites like eBay (www.ebay.com) and Freecycle (www.freecycle.org) are gold mines for perfectly excellent, previously used things. Please take pleasure in becoming the second (or third, or fourth) owner of something; it's a cost-effective and ecologically sustainable method to satisfy your demands.

Finally, purchasing less is the cornerstone of our minimalist lifestyles. Limiting our purchases to necessities is the most effective method to reduce the environmental impact of our consumption. We may assure that we, as people, are accountable for less resource depletion, human misery, and waste by doing so. If we genuinely do not require another sweater or pair of shoes, let us refrain from purchasing them for the sake of fashion. Consider the materials used to make them, the factories where they were produced, the cost of transporting them worldwide, and the eventual impact of their disposal. Let's base our purchase decisions on our requirements and the whole life cycle of a product—rather than the fact that we like the colour or saw it in an ad.

Let's reject being "consumers" and become "minsumers" instead. We will try to limit our consumption to what is necessary, reduce the impact of our consumption on the environment, and minimise the impact of our consumption on the lives of others.

If an extra benefit, such a mindset helps us in achieving our other minimalist goals: as we limit our consumption to save the environment, our living spaces will remain clean, tranquil, and clutter-free!

4

How You Can Start Living A Simpler Life - TODAY

WE'RE ready to put our new attitude into action now that we've developed our minimalist mindset. The **STREAMLINE** technique is described in detail in the following chapters: ten tried-and-true methods for getting rid of clutter and keeping it that way. They're simple to use and remember; each letter of the word signifies a different stage in our decluttering process. There will be no stopping us once we get them under our belts!

S - Start over

T - Trash, Treasure, or Transfer

R - Reason for each item

E - Everything in its place

A - All surfaces clear

M - Modules

L - Limits

I - If one comes in, one goes out

N - Narrow it down

E - Everyday maintenance

It's time to put our decluttering abilities to work! In the following chapter, we'll apply the STREAMLINE approach to individual rooms, addressing the difficulties and challenges that are unique to each. Feel free to jump around and begin wherever you like. Just because we discussed the rooms in a specific sequence doesn't imply you have to do the same. Start with the simplest, then the most difficult, then the smallest, then the largest—whatever appeals to you. So, let's get started on the minimalist makeover!

5

Your Home

The Living Room Or Family Room

THIS CHAPTER WILL CONCENTRATE on the living room (or what you may call your family room). It makes little difference how your walls are arranged—for our purposes, it is the space where family members assemble and guests congregate when they visit. It is the largest area in most houses and the one that sees the most action, so our decluttering efforts here will create a beautiful tone for the entire household.

S - Start over

However, before we begin, I'd like you to leave your residence. (It's right, you read that correctly.) Get to your feet, go out the door, and shut it behind you. Once you're outside, take a few moments to clear your mind and breathe in some fresh air. With our magical minimalist skills, we'll have decluttered your entire home by the time you return! Of course, I'm joking—but there is a point to this exercise.

Okay, you can go back inside now, but pretend you don't live there when you go through the front door. Enter with fresh eyes and an impartial perspective, as if you were a visitor. As if you were viewing your living environment for the first time from the perspective of a stranger. (It's a less arduous method to start again than dumping your living room into the front lawn.) So, how would you describe your initial impression? Do you like what you see? Is your living room calm and appealing, enticing you to stay? Or is it disorganised and overcrowded, making you want to escape? More specifically, if all of this wasn't yours, would you want to sit down and hang out in the centre of it?

We're rethinking our living spaces since clutter "disappears" when we become accustomed to it. We become accustomed to a coffee table that has been covered in periodicals, souvenirs, art supplies, and children's toys for weeks, months, or even years. We become accustomed to the laundry basket in the corner, the books heaped next to the sofa, and the DVDs packed around the television. We lose sight of the clutter; our viewpoint changes, and instead of looking at it, we gaze around it.

After you've analysed the overall picture, take a detailed look at the contents of the space. Examine every piece of furniture, every throw pillow, and every item. Is each of these products both helpful and beautiful? Do they appear to be in harmony with one another and appropriate in their respective settings? Or does it look like a flea market—or, worse, the inside of a storage unit? Would you bring it all back in if you emptied the contents onto your front yard, or would you be satisfied to evict a large portion?

Close your eyes and picture your perfect living room. Consider which pieces of furniture you'd keep and how you'd arrange them; consider what would be on your tables and shelves, as well as what would be in your drawers and cupboards. What distinguishes your fantasy room from your real one? Which things stayed and which disappeared completely? With a little decluttering, you may be able to turn your present area into your dream place.

T - Transfer, Treasure, or Trash?

First and foremost, let's get rid of the objects that didn't make it into your fantasy space. Because life is short, why put up with things that don't make you happy?

Start small and work your way up to greater responsibilities, according to common wisdom. Not a terrible concept, but let's try something different—something BIG. Your living room has some big objects and provides an excellent chance to begin with a boom. Purging just one piece of unneeded (or disliked) furniture can have a big impact—and it's a great motivator to go through the smaller stuff. It's as if that shabby old chair or orphan end table is a huge plugin, your clogged-up sink of stuff, and yanking it out clears the way for a deluge of clutter.

So prioritise your important tasks first. Is every piece of furniture used daily, or are certain pieces only there because "they always have been"? Think about how you and your family will use the space. Do you prefer the sofa or the floor? Is anyone ever seen sitting in the corner chair? Is the console helpful, or is it just a dumping ground for junk? Would having fewer pieces of furniture allow you to have more space for activities (lounging, playing games, gathering for a movie)?

Don't feel compelled to acquire certain goods just because they're expected (as in, "What would the neighbours say if we didn't have a recliner?"). If you have a big object you want to get rid of but are afraid of, take it out of the room for a few days. Put it in the basement or attic for the time being and see whether anyone misses it. Is its absence detrimental to your pleasure of the room, or does it improve it? Moving a piece out of the way may sometimes offer you a better perspective on it, and once it's out of the way, it's simpler to cut connections with it.

After you've dealt with the major objects, it's time to tackle the smaller ones, which, depending on the size of your living room, may be quite a number. The best approach is to take it one shelf at a time, drawer by drawer, pile by pile. (A single shelf doesn't seem so awful, does it?) Don't worry; we'll break things down into smaller, more doable jobs here.

Simply empty the contents (or throw them out) and organise them into Trash, Treasure, and Transfer piles. Clean up any collected rubbish (such as packaging, junk mail, and food wrappers), and place plates, glasses, and coffee cups in the sink. Go through your CD, DVD, and video game collections and donate those that have fallen out of favour. Remove any out-of-date magazines from the magazine rack. Examine hobby materials, board games, and books to ensure they are in "active" usage. Calculate the value of your knickknacks and ornamental objects and identify those that are genuinely Treasures (you know what to do with the others!).

Above all, please don't rush through it. Take the time to perform a thorough job, even if it means going through every single drawer for weeks or months. In the long term, such attentiveness will yield considerably bigger advantages.

R - Reason for each item

The living room may be a dumping ground for clutter due to its public character (and closeness to the front entrance). As a result, you'll need to be extra cautious that everything in the room belongs there. Remember, this is a living room, not a storage room: only items you (or your family) use daily should be kept in this area. Is there enough space for everyone to engage (in other words, is there enough space for genuine life) if you think of the room as a stage? Is the presence of too many props stifling the action?

As you go around the room, identify the purpose for each item's presence. The sofa, for example, is here because we sit on it to communicate, play games, and watch TV. The coffee table keeps our beverages and food and serves as a platform for pursuing our hobbies. We can watch movies together thanks to the DVD player. The mantel clock is a treasured family heirloom. The end table has a stack of magazines that no one ever reads. (Hmm...maybe we should do something about that one.) Don't simply look at the DVD collection or bookshelves while assessing the furnishings of your living room. Consider each thing separately, and consider if anybody still reads a certain book, watches a particular movie, or plays a particular game.

Consider each knickknack in turn, as you would with your décor. Do the ornamental objects in the space make you happy to look at? Or did they merely amass over time and serve no use other than to take up space? Clear the room of any non-functional items —sweep them from the shelves, mantle, console, and side tables. Put them in a box and go a week without using them. Extraneous objects can often limit our pleasure of a location without our even noticing it. When they're gone, we experience a surge of relief, as if we can finally stretch out and move around (without hitting or breaking anything). Take note of how family members and guests respond to the decluttered space—do they seem more at ease? Do they have greater freedom to roam around? Are they more eager to participate in activities?

Of course, if you genuinely miss an item—say, a souvenir from a memorable trip or a lovely handmade bowl—you are welcome to collect it from the box and return it to its proper location. If its presence makes you joyful, it has just as much purpose to be in the space as the necessary items. The trick is to choose and showcase only one or two of these treasures rather than transforming your living room into a gallery of them.

E - Everything in its proper position

Because the living area gets so much traffic, everything must have a place. Otherwise, things might quickly devolve into chaos!

As a result, establishing zones or activity areas is quite beneficial. Define the areas where you watch television, store movies, read magazines, play games, and use the computer. Make certain that the things associated with the activities are stored in their proper zone, and do everything possible to keep them from straying into another. DVDs should not be heaped on the coffee table; instead, they should have their own shelf or drawer. Similarly, magazines should not be placed on the screen, and toys should not be kept on the couch. Include all family members in creating the zones; this way; everyone will understand the system and share responsibility for its upkeep.

If the living room also serves as someone's office or craft space, confine the activity (and its associated accessories) to a clearly defined area. Set up a desk or worktable in a corner, against a wall, or at another location as far away from the main action of the room as feasible. If necessary, use a standing screen or a floor plant to create a visible (and psychological) border. The rationale for this is twofold: first, you don't want office materials pouring into the main living room. Second, you'll be a lot more productive if you don't have to clear toys from your desk before using them.

After you've divided the area into zones, allocate your belongings to the Inner Circle, Outer Circle, and Deep Storage. As you may recall, your Inner Circle products are those you utilise on a regular (or almost daily) basis. They should be stored in easily accessible areas, such as mid-level shelves and drawers near your activity zones. The remote control, current magazines, regularly used devices, and computer peripherals, and beloved books, CDs, DVDs, and games are all candidates for your living room's Inner Circle. Goods used less than once a week, such as hobby and craft supplies, reference books, and items for entertaining visitors, should be kept in your Outer Circle. These should be kept on upper and lower shelves and in less accessible drawers and cabinets. Seasonal decorations and items you value but can't now exhibit (maybe to toddler-proof the space) go in Deep Storage, preferably in the basement, attic, or another out-of-the-way location.

A - All surfaces clear

Could you put some refreshments on the coffee table if a neighbour came by right now? Is there anywhere for your kids to play a game or work on an art project? Or would either possibility be postponed (or abandoned) because you need to clean out too much clutter? Is there enough area on the floor for a little yoga, or would you get more of a workout shifting about furniture and other things to make some space?

Our living rooms are meant to be used for living. We are undermining the functioning of the room and cheating ourselves (and our families) out of extremely precious space if we treat them as improvised storage units and load them to the brim with things. Surfaces, such as the coffee table, side tables, worktable, or desk, are crucial. They are worthless for our present activities if carelessly stacked with periodicals, junk mail, toys, books, and incomplete craft projects. Similarly, if they are utilised as a display area for many trinkets, knickknacks, and other ornamental things, they impede the "living" in the room. Surfaces in the family room should not be designated for a lifeless parade of porcelain figurines but rather the contrary. They are intended for four-year-olds to paint, adolescents to play games with their friends, and adults to relax with a cup of coffee.

46

We should also try to maintain the floor (our largest surface) as uncluttered as possible. Children, in particular, want the room to roam, frolic, and explore; they should not be crammed into a little play area hidden behind wall-to-wall furniture and mountains of clutter. Adults benefit from a calm, clean environment as well. When we get home from a hard day at work, we need space to decompress, both emotionally and physically. We feel pressured, suffocated, and angry when we trip over items on our approach to the sofa or gaze about at a jumble of material. When the room is bare and neat, on the other hand, we have plenty of space—and peace of mind—to sit back, relax, and breathe. As a result, make an effort to gather loose things and keep them out of the way of children.

To use a business word, we should conceive of our living rooms as "flex space." In an office, flex space is a work area that anybody may use. When an employee comes to work in the morning, he takes a seat at an open (empty) desk for the day. When he departs in the evening, he takes all of his things with him, freeing up the desk for someone else to use the next day. Our living spaces should work in the same way: the floor and surfaces should be vacant, ready to accommodate the day's activities, and when those activities end, they should be emptied of all objects, leaving them open and ready for the next person to use.

M - Modules

In the broadest sense, each room is a container that stores everything associated with its purpose. However, because our living room (like many of our other rooms) serves several roles, things may quickly get disorganised. As a result, we divided it into zones, establishing separate spaces for different activities. Now we'll take it a step further and create modules, which will consolidate particular things for specific activities.

Create modules in your living room for your various collections, such as CDs, DVDs, and video games. Rather than keeping them in a confusing mess, separate them and assign a particular shelf, drawer, or container to each group. Consolidating similar things allows us to readily detect duplicates, filter out undesirables, and understand the extent of our collections. It also assists other family members and us return items to their designated locations, keeping them from straying across the room or into other sections of the house. Make the same arrangements for books (on designated shelves), magazines (on a shelf or rack), and electrical and computer devices (in a special drawer, cabinet, or container).

Modules are very handy for storing craft and hobby items. Instead of storing them all in the same drawer or cabinet, organise them by activity: knitting, scrapbooking, painting, model building, jewellery making, and so on. Assign a container to each task; transparent plastic storage bins and the hefty cardboard boxes in which reams of paper are sold work nicely (cover them with fabric or contact paper to make them more attractive). Deep, rectangular baskets may also work. When you're ready to start a new pastime, just extract its module and unpack its materials onto a suitable (clear!) surface. Just place everything back into the container and return it to its designated storage location when you're done. Modules efficiently maintain the living room's flex area by making it easy to move stuff away.

Consider the following scenario: your family has finished dinner and has gone to the living room. When the kids want to watch a favourite movie, they just pull it from the DVD module and place it in the player; there's no mad rush under the sofa, behind the bookcases, or amid the CDs and video games (and no one is accused of "having it last"). Your husband settles down with a magazine, grabbing the latest edition off the rack without having to sift through mounds of junk. And you decide to do some scrapbooking, taking your supplies from a neighbouring cabinet and arranging them on the empty coffee table. After the evening, the DVD is returned to its bin, the magazine to its rack, and your craft items to their container. The living area is already clear for the next day's events, with everything, tucked away in its modules!

L - Limits

As minimalists, we want to limit our collections to our favourite objects; otherwise, they tend to expand uncontrollably, and before we realise it, we're overrun with stuff. Limits can be set as either a certain number or a specific quantity of space. For example, when it comes to books, you may opt to limit your collection to one hundred or the amount of space available on your bookshelf. In either case, you're limiting the overall number and ensuring that your library only contains your favourite and most often read books.

Set restrictions on every sort of item in your living room, including books, CDs, DVDs, and games. Once you've achieved them, it's time to get rid of the old and make room for the new. Our tastes evolve with time; we become weary of movies, music, and activities we once enjoyed. Yet, for some reason, we frequently keep these out-of-date objects, whether out of guilt for the money spent or in the hope that we would rediscover an interest in them. Instead of keeping them permanently, go through them regularly and donate the ones you no longer use. A new, pared-down collection is far more enjoyable to peruse than an indiscriminate array of titles. Borrow from the library instead of buying if you desire novelty; this way, you may enjoy a broad range of entertainment without the stress (or price) of ownership.

In the case of hobby and craft supplies, your modules set a natural limit on the number of materials you may have on hand. If they're at capacity, don't add to them until you've depleted your present supply—either by tackling planned tasks, finishing unfinished ones, or just cleaning out what you don't intend to use. Imposing limitations provides you with the perfect reason to get rid of undesirable items (such the chartreuse yarn, chintzy beads, or poor cloth) that might diminish your excitement for the work at hand. Choose your favourites and toss the others!

Also, keep your collections to a minimum. I'm not sure if the desire to collect is inherent in human nature, but most of us have accumulated items simply for the sake of collecting, whether it's baseball cards, Beanie Babies, vintage teacups, first edition books, movie memorabilia, commemorative coins, foreign stamps, or antique nutcrackers. We like the thrill of the search and the pleasure of discovering a new item to add to our collection (the rarer, the better).

Unfortunately, the Internet (particularly eBay) has made finding such "treasures" far too simple. Previously, our collections were hampered by a lack of availability and access; we had to trawl antique stores and flea markets for fresh treasures. A universe of "things" is now at our fingertips; we may acquire a collection that formerly took years to develop in a matter of hours online! As a result, we must place our own restrictions on collections, limiting our purchases to a set quantity rather than buying everything we can discover.

Finally, place restrictions on your decorative objects. Take cues from traditional Japanese houses, where just one or two carefully selected objects are on show at a time. Instead of competing for attention with a dozen other objects, you may respect and appreciate those most significant to you in this way. That doesn't mean you have to get rid of the rest of your decorations (unless, of course, you want to). Simply construct a "décor module" to house your favourite items; bring them out for exhibition a few at a time, and rotate them throughout the year. It will give your space a new appearance and put your treasures in the limelight.

I - If one comes in, one goes out

While we gradually clean our living spaces, we must ensure that nothing new enters. We can assure a zero net gain of items by following the One In-One Out rule, which requires us to offset each entering item with a departing one.

Unlike the occasional pruning of our collections, this technique necessitates quick choice and action. If we bring home a new book, game, or DVD, we must immediately discard an old one. As a result, rather than increasing in quantity, our collection improves in quality. Why keep a movie (or book) that you just saw (or read) once and didn't particularly enjoy? Don't allow it to take up valuable space; instead, replace it with something new and interesting. Make this a habit, and your living room will be transformed from a bland tribute to previous hobbies and pastimes to a vibrant place reflecting your family's present inclinations.

Similarly, when a new edition of a magazine arrives, throw the old ones in the recycling bin (or pass it on to friends or relatives). If you haven't found the time to open it, you're probably not interested in the content. At the absolute least, rapidly scan it and take out interesting articles; a few sheets of paper in your reading pile are less intimidating than a whole issue. In addition, if you sign up for a new subscription, you should cancel an existing one. We may have many hobbies, but we only have so much time in the day; choose just one or two magazines so that you can devote enough time to them. You may always exchange them for fresh ones the next year.

Apply the same principle to hobbies and crafts. Again, our free time is limited; instead of pursuing every passing interest, focus on one or two activities about which you are genuinely passionate. If you adopt a new activity, give up an old one that no longer interests you—it will free up your time and space. Perhaps you've lost interest in jewellery making but would like to learn to play the guitar; abandon the former to pursue the latter. Sell any remaining materials on Craigslist or eBay, or donate them to a nearby school.

The One In-One Out guideline also applies to décor. Assume you're out shopping and something catches your attention. You believe it's ideal for your house and imagine you'd get a lot of joy from gazing at it every day. However, as a minimalist, you pause (and rightfully so)—do you really want to add another thing into your home? If the item is truly unique, you don't have to deny yourself its visual pleasure—as long as you contribute something in exchange. You want to avoid acquiring more; nevertheless, replacing anything you have with something better is not forbidden. If you determine that the new object is not worthy of such a sacrifice, it is preferable to pass on it and wait for something more deserving to come along.

N - NARROW it down

It's nice to have a constant state of things, but narrowing it down is even better (and essential to developing a minimalist lifestyle). In an ideal world, we would own nothing more than what we require.

A living room must have some type of seating for family members at a bare minimum. Extreme minimalists (from non-Western cultures) may be quite satisfied with only a few floor cushions. A lounge chair may suffice for a bachelor. A sofa, on the other hand, may be considered necessary by a family. Do the math: if your home only has three people, do you really need furniture that seats eight? You can easily improvise some foldable seats (or create a fun, bohemian atmosphere by lounging on the floor). Consider the furniture's footprint as well; I've seen overstuffed, enormous sectionals that practically filled the entire room. Is the "comfort" of such a beast worth the floor space it consumes? Could you satisfy your seating requirements with something smaller and slimmer?

Let's move on to the topic of tables. Again, most living rooms will necessitate at least one table to suit the activities of the family. A simple coffee table may be sufficient. If the room is also used as an office or craft area, an extra desk or worktable may be required. Anything beyond that, on the other hand, is frequently just ornamental. Consider if you truly need the end tables, side tables, console tables, and other present tables in the space. If the primary purpose of the end table is to hold a magazine and the remote control, consider reassigning that duty to the coffee table to save space. Do the same with the console table that serves no use other than to exhibit your ornaments; get rid of the knickknacks, and you no longer need the table. Wow! All-out decluttering in one fell swoop!

Investing in multi-functional furniture is another approach to "narrow it down." As previously said, a sleeper sofa may double as both your family's couch and a guest bed. A coffee table with built-in drawers or cabinets can remove the need for additional storage and free up valuable floor space. The same is true for ottomans: if you're going to have one, have it serve double duty by storing some of your belongings. Such items give maximal usefulness with a small footprint, giving us more room to move around.

Your living room may also have a television and gadgets entertainment centre. But consider this: do you need the TV? As surprising as it may seem, many people live wonderfully satisfying, amusing, and educated lives without one. The Internet is a great source of news, and if you have a broadband connection, you can watch a variety of shows online. I'm not asking you to stop watching TV today; I'm merely offering the concept as an option. Consider it (or turn it off for a week and see if you miss it). When you think about it, you might conclude that's not such a horrible idea—and when your existing set dies, you might decide not to replace it. The added benefit is that if you don't have a TV, you don't need a cabinet, stand, or another piece of furniture to hold it. (Alternatively, you can avoid the stand entirely by attaching the TV to the wall.)

Most of our living rooms also feature shelves where we keep books, magazines, games, CDs, DVDs, hobby supplies, knickknacks, and so on. All I can say is that the less you have, the less storage you need—so start pruning those collections! Develop hobbies that require little resources, such as singing, origami, or learning a new language, and play games that use a tiny deck of cards rather than enormous boards and hundreds of plastic pieces. Use innovative ways to satisfy your entertainment requirements, such as borrowing goods from friends or the library rather than purchasing them. (It's pointless to own something you're just going to read, watch, or listen to once.)

Consider going digital for those titles you want to own. Instead of purchasing DVDs, download movies from the Internet. Convert your music to MP3 files and buy it in that format in the future; not only will it decrease your clutter, but you'll have access to your collection (through an iPod or MP3 device) anywhere you go. Invest in an electronic reader and purchase digital books rather than physical ones. A single paperback-sized device may contain hundreds of titles (and provide access to thousands more), obviating the need for whole bookshelves.

Use technology to reduce the size of your photo albums as well. Instead of keeping those heavy books, scan the contents and convert them to digital format. You can print the ones you want to show one at a time as they come to mind. There are several advantages to using digital photos. For starters, they are significantly easier to obtain. If you want to look at photos from your vacation to Paris or the workplace Christmas party, you may do it on your computer. (You may not bother if you had to search through a closet or shoebox to find them.) Second, they're considerably easier to distribute. Emailing your friends fresh photos of your baby or trip is faster, more convenient, and less expensive than sending printed copies via the mail (or wait for them to visit and look through your albums). Third, paper pictures can degrade over time or be destroyed in a flood, fire, or other natural calamities. Because digital photographs may be kept in numerous locations (on a hard drive, online, and various DVDs), you are less likely to lose those important images.

E - EVERYDAY MAINTENANCE

Because there is so much going on in the living room, we must always be aware of what is going on. Devoting some time to daily upkeep is well worth the effort; you and your family will have a far more comfortable environment in which to relax and enjoy one other's company.

Of course, we must always be prepared with our protection shields. This area is only a few steps from the entrance door and is frequently the first place entering items rest. (In fact, some of them appear to be locked here indefinitely!) Keep an eye out for invaders. (What's in the box next to the door? Who is the person whose jacket is lying over the couch? Is that a piece of junk mail on the coffee table?) When you see anything that doesn't belong, don't just throw up your hands in despair and recline on the couch; fight back. Flush such intruders out at first sight, and make certain that nothing entering or passing through the room has a chance to halt. Hang up jackets, put shoes away, handle mail, and transport new goods immediately to their designated locations.

Keep an eye out for areas where clutter tends to accumulate, such as the coffee table, end table, or other surfaces in the room. Take dishes, glasses, and leftover food to the kitchen as soon as you finish your snack. After you've finished a game or a creative activity, put all supplies in their modules and tuck them away. Please encourage your children to return all toys to their proper places once they have played with them. Clutter has little chance of accumulating if you straighten up after every activity. Furthermore, if you come across any stray things when vacuuming or dusting, don't just clean around them; tidy them up!

To make matters worse, the living area is where you're most likely to come across other people's clutter. Ideally, this issue will fade over time as members of the household learn to respect the flex area and take personal belongings with them when they leave the room. In the meanwhile, you may have to roll up your sleeves, dig in, and boomerang that item back to its rightful owners. Make a routine of going through the space each evening before bed and clearing it of anything that doesn't belong. It just takes a few minutes, yet it makes a tremendous impact. You may nag, preach, and talk about keeping things clean until you're blue in the face, but the greatest way to motivate people is to set a good example.

Finally, keep decluttering regularly—unless you're already a minimalist expert, there's always something else you can get rid of. Scan your books, CDs, and DVDs regularly for items you no longer desire; something you loved last month (or even last week) may no longer be appealing to you. If you find an old magazine, throw it away; if you've gotten tired of particular hobbies, get rid of the supplies; and if any object has a coating of dust on it, really consider letting it go. Please keep it simple, keep it fresh, and keep it calm in your living area!

Bedroom

We'll work our minimalist magic in the bedroom in this chapter. More than any other in the house, this room should be a sanctuary of calm and tranquillity amid our hurried life. As a result, we have some significant work ahead of us, but once we're done, we'll have the ideal setting for a well-deserved relaxation.

S - Start over

Your bedroom should be the cleanest space in your home. It serves an extremely vital purpose: it provides consolation for your tired spirit after a long day of work, school, childcare, housecleaning, and whatever else you manage to cram into your day. It should be a place of rest for your body as much as your mind.

Close your eyes for a few seconds and imagine your perfect bedroom. Consider every element as if it were a magazine layout:

- The bed design.
- The colour of the sheets, duvet, and blanket.

- The pillows, lighting, flooring, décor, and other furniture in the room.

What type of mood is it in? (I think it's not chaotic.) Is it a peaceful haven? A romantic getaway? An opulent suite? Although I don't know your own likes, one thing is certain: there isn't a speck of clutter in your ideal space. And rightfully so: it's difficult to feel pampered when you're buried in things, and a storage facility isn't exactly romantic.

To start over, remove everything from the room except the bed. This piece of furniture can stay because, by definition, the room is for sleeping (and we don't want to throw our backs out). Empty it down to its basic bones and temporarily store everything in a neighbouring room. Similarly, leave any large, wardrobe-related objects that you will undoubtedly maintain, such as an armoire or dresser, in place. For the time being, however, everything else must go: desks, tables, chairs, storage boxes, laundry bins, potted plants, treadmills, ab crunchers, televisions, laptops, lights, books, magazines, vases, knickknacks, and so on.

Now sit down on the bed and take a look around. Isn't it a big difference? You probably have no idea how much room you have. Is it more open, calm, and relaxing now? Is it simpler to stretch, clear your thoughts, and breathe now? That's exactly how a bedroom should feel! It should revitalise and revive you rather than stress you out and make you exhausted. The best thing is that you don't need an interior designer or a costly makeover to create this lovely ambience. You only need to declutter!

T - Transfer, Treasure, or Trash?

Make your Trash, Treasure, and Transfer piles and begin going through the items of your bedroom. Don't worry about clothing or accessories just yet; it's a separate task that we'll cover in a later chapter. For the time being, focus on anything else, especially things that have nothing to do with sleeping or dressing.

You're likely to run into an intriguing dilemma here: you'll come across objects that don't belong in any of those heaps. You don't want to throw them away or put them in the Transfer pile to sell or give away; in fact, you'd like to retain them. However, they cannot be placed in your bedroom's Treasure pile because they are unrelated to sleep or clothes. The issue is that while the goods may exist in your life, they do not belong in your bedroom.

Unfortunately, our bedrooms frequently serve as overflow drains for our belongings. When a sink becomes overflowing, the surplus water sloshes into the hole at the rear of the basin; similarly, when our living spaces get overflowing, the spillover material leaks through our bedroom doors. Assume you have visitors arriving in an hour and are hurriedly cleaning the living and dining rooms. You've packed everything you can into the closets and drawers, but you'll eventually run out of room. So, what are you going to do? Keep the extras in the bedroom. At the very least, you may close the door and hide it from view when entertaining. But, all too frequently, that refugee stuff settles in there, and before you know it, you're using your bedroom as an impromptu solution to your clutter problem.

Feel free to rename your Transfer pile "Transfer Out of the Room" and put anything that goes elsewhere in the home in it. This pile may include everything from periodicals to children's toys to your rowing machine. You could even want to include some mementoes and emotional things in the mix. However, be certain that the objects contained within have a proper position someplace. You don't want to drag a mound of homeless garbage from room to room. If an item's role is so ambiguous that you don't know where to put it, the ideal location for it may be in your contribution box.

R - Reason for everything

Our bedrooms' primary role is to provide space for sleeping and clothing storage. As a result, when we ask the resident items what their reason for being there, the response must be related to leisure, relaxation, or wardrobe—otherwise, they may risk deportation.

Your bed is probably smug right now, knowing it will pass this test with flying colours. The items on your nightstand, vanity, or dresser may be a bit tenser, but some of them have every right to be there. The alarm clock, glasses, Toilet tissue, and the book you're now reading are all secure. You might retain the vase of flowers and a few candles—they're perfect for creating a romantic and relaxed mood. A few additional things may get access to this desired, snug space—but to be honest, I can't think of many. "Because there is nowhere for them to go" is not a valid argument to keep them here!

Now, let's talk about the items that don't belong here yet frequently attempt to get in. For example, take that annoying laundry basket; sure, the bed makes a wonderful surface for folding clothes—but do it and be done with it immediately! If it's gathering your next load, locate another location for it. Nothing kills the mood faster than a pile of dirty socks while you're having a spontaneous, romantic evening with your partner. The same is true for your toddler's toys; it's difficult to get things going when a swarm of stuffed animals surrounds you.

Another concern is the lack of craft supplies. When they can't find refuge elsewhere, they frequently move to this room. Unless you're knitting in your sleep, yarn and needles should be kept out of the bedroom. If it's a pre-bedtime activity, we'll make an exception; in that case, put everything in a box or bag and tuck it beneath the bed, and I won't complain. Just don't transform your boudoir into a fully-stocked craft shop, if only for the sake of your lover. Similarly, choose another location to store gym equipment and computer supplies; hand weights and hard drives are not appealing!

Perhaps I don't give knickknacks a fair trial, but I believe they have no place in the bedroom. A few exceptional items are fine, but consider if you need fifteen of them lined up across your dresser. A room full of trinkets might feel stale and museum-like, and if you make the wrong move, you can break something delicate. Furthermore, the more things on your surfaces, the more difficult it is to clean them—and who wants to spend any extra time on housework?

E - Everything in its proper place

Everything in our bedrooms must have a place if we want them to be calm and serene. When things are tucked away, there is a sense of serenity; scattered materials, on the other hand, disrupt our peaceful environment.

It's simple to define zones in the bedroom—you'll need one for sleeping and one for dressing. You may also have a grooming zone (for putting on cosmetics, fixing your hair, and so on), especially if you share a bathroom with other members of your household. I don't recommend having an office zone in the bedroom unless you have no other option; in that case, do all you can to keep it distinct from the main space. It's tough to go asleep when your desk is stacked high with work, bills, and anything else that causes you to worry. Install a screen or hang a curtain to conceal it while not in use.

The Inner Circle of your bedroom should include objects you use every day, such as the aforementioned alarm clock, reading glasses, grooming products, and in-season clothes. Of course, instead of being strewn over the room, they should all be in their proper locations. Clothes should be stored in closets and dressers rather than heaped on the floor or thrown over chairs. Make it a practice to fold, hang, or put your clothing in the hamper as soon as you remove it. Cosmetics should be kept in a makeup bag or container, and other accessories, such as shoes, belts, purses, and jewellery, should have a specific space in your closet or drawers. The contents of your Inner Circle should be accessible—but not necessarily visible.

Keep additional linens and out-of-season clothes in your Outer Circle. Keep them in difficult-to-reach nooks and crannies, such as beneath the bed (everyone's favourite storage location), lower dresser drawers, and higher shelves in closets and armoires. But keep in mind that your Outer Circle isn't a catch-all for things you don't know what to do with; items must be utilised at least a few times a year to qualify for this space. If you have orphan pillowcases, your adult son's childhood sheets, or a duvet cover that no longer matches your décor, it's time to declutter.

I can't think of a single bedroom item that would be ideal for deep storage. Garages, attics, and basements are not ideal places to store bedding; moreover, any bedding you own should be rotated regularly in your family. Even seasonal linens (such as flannel sheets and thick blankets) are improper for such an out-of-the-way storage location. Simply pick what goes in your Inner and Outer Circles, and you're finished! That makes it easier, doesn't it?

A - All surfaces clear

Let's begin with the essential surface in this space: the bed! There should be no ifs, and, or buts about it. Because your bed is vital to your health and well-being and is used for at least a quarter of the day, it should always be ready to perform its intended function.

Keep the beautiful throw pillows and other non-essentials to a minimum because your bed is a practical surface, not a decorative one. It's a chore to make the bed each night, and the fewer items you have to tidy, organise and worry with, the better. Keep it simple, like luxury hotels: crisp white sheets and pillows covered with a soft duvet make for a lovely, minimalist retreat—no accessories required! Just keep in mind that when I say the bed is a useful surface, I don't mean it should fulfil every purpose imaginable; it's not supposed to be your washing station, office, or kids' play area. If it occurs to fulfil one of these functions briefly, remove the clothing, paperwork, or children's toys as soon as possible.

Of course, the bed isn't the only surface that has to be watched. The more furniture you have—nightstands, vanities, dressers, and tables—the more alert you must be (another good reason to have less furniture!). Don't allow these objects to collect stray goods such as clothing, mail, spare cash, cosmetics, and DVDs. Clear off their tops and save them for the few items that belong there. If you've confined some trinkets to the bedroom because they're not "good enough" for your living area, think about whether they're "good enough" to maintain at all.

Last but not least, don't overlook the floor. Get rid of those stacks of books and magazines (how many can you read at once, anyway?) and anything else that has gathered while you were distracted. Above important, don't let any garments go underfoot and create a pile. When you start a "floordrobe," you have a far greater problem; a rising mountain of clothing isn't healthy for your environment or your clothes! The only place on the floor where you may put things is beneath the bed. Use but do not misuse this important storage area; in other words, do not use it to hide junk.

M - Modules

If you don't have a linen closet elsewhere in the house, store your excess bedding in the bedroom using modules. Under-the-bed plastic bins are ideal for keeping extra sheets, pillows, and blankets. Separate them by season, so you don't have to rummage among flannels and heavy comforters to find your cool summer linens. Do the same in each of your bedrooms; keep the kids' and guests' linens hidden beneath their mattresses in their modules. Therefore, each individual will have fast and easy access to their bedding, avoiding the clutter that may occur when they are all heaped together on a shelf.

Consolidating your linens also allows you to see how many you have. When we are not looking, sheets appear to multiply. We buy a new set every so often because we want a new appearance, our old ones look outdated, or visitors are on their way, with little regard for those we already own. The old ones are put to a "just in case" bin, and our collection continues to expand with each passing year. When you add them all up, you might be surprised at how many you have! Putting them into modules allows you to reduce the number of them to a manageable number.

Make modules for grooming products if you store them in the bedroom. Cosmetics, combs, hairbrushes, and styling items should be kept in a compact bag or container that may be hidden while not in use. Why show off your full beauty arsenal to your partner (or overnight guests)? It's better to keep a little mystery than to destroy a romantic setting with a slew of hairspray, foot powder, or deodorant on your dresser. You could also want to dedicate a small tray, box, or drawer for the items that come out of your pockets daily, such as your wallet, loose change, transport cards, keys, and so on. Consolidating them makes them seem neater and much simpler to discover the next morning. Books, magazines, craft projects, and other pre-bedtime diversions benefit from a little modular organising as well, making them easy to tuck away and slide under the bed as you start to doze off.

L - Limits

To create and maintain a tranquil mood in the bedroom, use limitations freely. The less clutter you see, the more tranquil you will feel, which might be the difference between a restless or restful night's sleep.

First and foremost, keep the amount of furnishings in the space to a minimum. You don't have to buy (or retain) all of the matching pieces in a bedroom set just because it includes six of them. Instead of cramming the entire ensemble into the space, choose only the parts you require. Seating (such as seats or benches) should be limited to the number of individuals sharing the space, and clothing storage (such as armoires or dressers) should be limited to one per person. The latter results in a more simplified wardrobe and a more spacious bedroom. Limiting the contents of your furnishings aids in the reduction of the furnishings themselves.

Second, keep the visible items to a minimum. Keep no more than three objects on your nightstand or top of your dresser, for example. This method emphasises beautiful objects while leaving plenty of room for useful ones. Don't allow a jumble of hairspray bottles or a lovely vase on your vanity to compete for attention with a pile of magazines. Similarly, don't put yourself in a position where you'll knock over knickknacks when reaching for your snooze clock.

Third, reduce the number of linens you own to a specific number. Two sets of sheets per bed are usually plenty and can be changed according to your washing schedule. Set your limit based on your household's needs; if you have regular overnight guests or potty-training children, you may need a few more. In the case of blankets and quilts, climate also plays a factor; a family in Cornwall will not require as many as a family in the Scottish Highlands. In general, don't store more than your family (and visitors) can utilise at any given moment. A pleasant home is defined by its inhabitants' warmth, love, and hospitality, not by the number of duvets stashed away in the linen closet.

I - If one comes in, one goes out

Take control of the things that come into your bedroom as you declutter them. You don't want to delete ten items just to discover that you've collected double that amount in the interim. Make it a habit to remove an old object whenever a new one enters the room.

Linen stashes necessitate extra caution. For some reason, when we purchase a new sheet set, blanket, quilt, or duvet, we are frequently hesitant to discard the old. The need to keep extra bedding appears to be hard-wired into our DNA. Perhaps we're frightened of losing electricity in the middle of winter and needing to layer it on to remain warm, or we anticipate a dozen unexpected overnight visitors will show up at our door; or we believe they'll come in useful the next time we're moving, painting, or having a picnic. There are only so many linens we'll ever need, no matter how we explain it, and keeping them for some hypothetical circumstance in the future is taking up some very real space right now. Keep the One In-One Out guideline in mind, and the next time you buy new bedding, give the old—and think of the warmth and comfort you're offering someone else.

Applying the same logic to anything that enters the bedroom will make decluttering much easier. Rather of adding more, refresh your décor by changing or rotating things. (Store extras in a décor module and rotate them regularly.) If you bring in fresh bedtime reading, you should either dispose of the old one or return it to its proper location. Instead of cramming a new piece of furniture into the room, exchange it for something comparable. (If you believe you "need" it to hold more stuff, first simplify it!) If you stick to this method, you'll be able to keep clutter out of your sleeping area.

N - Narrow it down

One of my favourite steps is "narrow it down" since this is when the true minimalist fun begins! Nowhere is this more entertaining or socially acceptable than in the bedroom! I've always been a touch anti-establishment, and violating the norms of consumer (or decorative) correctness is my way of "sticking it to the man."

Our bedrooms are our universes. Few outsiders visit this personal place, and those that do are already familiar with us (and thus won't criticise us based on our furniture, or lack thereof). As a result, we may freely indulge our minimalist dreams here, without regard for societal conventions. Doesn't it seem like fun? It may be unpleasant to sit guests on the floor in your living room, but nobody knows (or cares) if you sleep on it in your bedroom.

Look for ways to reduce your linen usage as well. Consider if separate winter and summer bedding is essential; plain cotton will suffice all year in most regions. Similarly, select a duvet cover that will function in all seasons; avoid heavy velvet, for example, favour something more flexible. You may decrease the contents of your linen closet without compromising comfort by making sensible selections. Instead of collecting sheets for an army, limit your collection to what is really necessary—whether it is two sets per bed or just one. If you don't have many overnight guests, your guest linens can serve as a backup set.

E - Everyday maintenance

Although the bedroom may not see as much traffic as other areas of the house, it still needs regular upkeep to maintain it clean and clutter-free.

The first item on the list is to make the bed every day! This simple activity takes only a few minutes to accomplish, yet it can totally change the space and set the tone for the rest of the day. A freshly made bed is one of life's small joys, beckoning you to sink into it and unwind after a long day's work. It also emanates peace and order and has a strong impact on keeping the bedroom nice and orderly. When the bed is undone, a shambles in the rest of the room doesn't seem out of place; everything just appears to be a wreck. When your bedding is perfectly smoothed, tucked, and folded, the clutter has no hiding place and is far less likely to accumulate.

Secondly, search the room for misplaced clothing. When we remove a jacket, sweater, or pair of stockings, especially when we are getting ready to go to bed after a hard day, the item does not always return to its proper place.

Put away any stray items as soon as you notice them.

Don't put off the work till "later"; by then, more items will have been added, and the chore will have expanded.

Shoes and bags, in particular, may be difficult to keep track of; these things enjoy going out on the town, and you'll often find a swarm of them waiting at the door. Allow them to have their unique spot in the closet (to which they must return each night), so they don't take up floor space in your area of the room. Properly storing clothes and accessories—on hangers and shelves, rather than in heaps on the floor—produces a more durable wardrobe and a more pleasant atmosphere.

Third, keep an eye out for unwelcome "guests" in the bedroom. Even in such a secluded setting, certain things manage to find their way in (usually in the arms of other family members). If you find your toddler's stuffed toy or your spouse's tennis racket hiding in the corner, don't invite it to spend the night; instead, boomerang it straight back where it belongs. Similarly, once you've finished reading that mystery novel or viewing your favourite romantic comedy on DVD, don't leave it by your bedside. Return it to its proper module in the living room or office, unless you have a book-shelf in your bedroom. Clear the room before closing your eyes, and you'll wake up to a lovely, tranquil environment every morning!

Wardrobe

It's time to deal with the mess in our closets. One of the great delights of being a minimalist is having a simplified wardrobe! This chapter is for you if you have a lot of clothing but nothing to wear. We'll look at how simplifying our wardrobe may save us time, money, space, and stress—all while making it simpler to appear well-dressed.

S - Start over

Cleaning out your closet does not have to be a hassle; in fact, it can be a lot of fun! It is, in fact, one of my favourite decluttering hobbies. The process is undoubtedly easier than handling a full room: there is no furniture to consider, tchotchkes to consider, or other people's belongings to deal with. To be honest, I think of it as "me time" rather than "cleaning time." I like to throw on some music, pour myself a drink of wine, and put on my fashion show while I go through my closet. Purging dowdy old clothes and designing fantastic new ensembles is a pleasant couple of hours, and having additional closet space at the end is a lovely reward.

To Start Over, remove everything out of your closet, drawers, armoire, and anywhere else you keep your clothes and spread it out on your bed. And when I say everything, I mean everything! Reach into those dark corners and bring out your sister's wedding bell-bottoms, bubble skirt, and bridesmaid outfit. Dive into the back corners for those cowboy boots, platform sandals, and strappy stilettos you've never been able to wear. Remove all of your under-wear, socks, pyjamas, and pantyhose from their drawers and line up your purses for examination. Continue until you're left with nothing but empty drawers, barren shelves, and naked hangers.

But before we go any farther, let us pause for a moment of intro-spection. To develop a minimalist wardrobe, we must first under-stand what works best for us, since when we have a restricted amount of clothing, they must all do their part. So, think about your style: is it classic, athletic, preppy, punk, bohemian, glamorous, vintage, romantic, or modern? Consider your preferred colours: do you prefer light pastels, dark jewel tones, or bright primary colours? Do you look better in close-fitting clothing or free and flowing ones? Do you prefer natural materials like cotton and wool or high-tech fabrics like polyester blends? When you examine your clothes, keep your responses in mind; items that don't match your style or prefer-ences are more likely to spend time in your closet than on your body.

Consider the following scenario: a fire, flood, or other calamity has destroyed your whole wardrobe, and you must reconstruct it from the ground up. (Yikes!) Because your resources are limited, you must make wise decisions. Consider the absolute necessities you'd require to get through a normal week. Socks, underwear, one or two pairs of pants, a couple of shirts, a jacket, a multipurpose pair of shoes, and maybe a sweater, skirt, and pair of pantyhose or tights. Choose pieces that are acceptable for both work and play and that can be layered to keep you comfortable in various climates. You must mix and match them and put together a range of ensembles with only a few items. This activity highlights your most useful clothing items and serves as a solid basis for your minimalist wardrobe.

You may create your ideal wardrobe once you've determined your key necessities as well as your preferred styles, colours, fabrics, and shapes. The best thing is that you get to be your stylist! Keep in mind the image you want to create as you go through your clothes —cool professional, elegant bohemian, Ivy League prepster—and choose (and reject) things accordingly. Keep the dresses and avoid the dowdy sweats if you want a more elegant image. If you're working your way up the corporate ladder, pencil skirts are preferable over peasant shirts. Be the curator of your wardrobe: choose products that complement your style and help you look and feel your best.

T - Transfer, Treasure, or Trash?

Try everything on now that it's out of your closet. How do you know that cocktail dress or three-piece suit still fits if you haven't worn it in five years? Do a three-sixty or two in front of the mirror after putting on each item. We're all aware that just because something appears nice on a hanger doesn't imply it will look good on us, and, conversely, an item that seems dreary on its own may spring to life when we put it on. Mix and match individual pieces throughout your fashion show: experiment with different combinations and discover out precisely what matches with what. You'll discover your most attractive and adaptable pieces of clothes as a result of this approach.

Make your Trash, Treasure, and Transfer piles and prepare yourself for some tough decisions. It's a good idea to keep your castoffs in boxes or garbage bags, not because you intend to toss them away, but because it keeps them out of sight. As a result, once you've chosen to discard an object, your decision will be "final"; your gaze will not be drawn to it again, enticing you to recover it from the reject pile. Take a pause and re-read the philosophy chapters if your determination begins to waver; sometimes, all you need is a little pep talk to steel your will and keep you going!

Put everything in your Trash pile that is beyond repairs (or your ability or desire to do so), such as the blouse with the stubborn wine stain, the shirt with the frayed collar, the pants with the worn-out knees, the skirt with the large tear, the threadbare jacket, the stockings with runs, the stretched-out undies, the socks without mates, and the sweaters with undeniable holes. If you can't reach inside it, put it on, and wear it in public, it doesn't belong in your closet. Of course, this does not imply that these items will end up in a landfill. All the better if you can recycle or reuse them (maybe as dust cloths). However, only retain them if you have a specific need in mind.

Decluttering would be a breeze if we just had to deal with worn-out stuff! Unfortunately, most of our garments outlive their usefulness before they are replaced. As a result, make excellent use of your Transfer pile; it's for all of those perfectly nice clothing that are no longer suitable for you. Put it here if it doesn't fit or isn't flattering, if it's outdated or inappropriate, or if you've simply gotten tired of it. Include any clothing that makes you feel self-conscious, uncomfortable, or out of place—you know, the ones you take off minutes after putting them on. Don't let this dreck pile up in your closet. They obstruct your nice stuff, perplex you when you're getting dressed, and make you feel as if you have nothing to wear.

While some pieces may be completely inappropriate for you, they may be ideal for someone else. Instead of letting them rot in your closet, give them a second chance. If you still have the tags on an item, ask if you can return it—most stores will take unworn items for a reasonable period (typically thirty to ninety days) after purchase. Otherwise, consider selling it on eBay or in a consignment store; major brands and designer items may bring in a tidy sum. Alternatively, you may give your clothes to a thrift store or a nonprofit organisation like Dress for Success; in exchange, you'll receive a clean closet, some good karma, and possibly even a tax write-off.

Work your way through the following steps to identify your Treasures, and you'll have a minimalist wardrobe in no time. If you like to go more slowly, here's an almost simple alternate approach. Obtain three spools of ribbon: one green, one yellow, and one red. Tie a bow around the hanger after you've worn it: green if it made you feel great, red if it made you feel frumpy, and yellow if you're undecided. Keep the greens and yellows as Treasures after six months, and Trash or Transfer the reds. If you don't have a ribbon on something, it indicates you haven't worn it at all—and you know where it belongs!

R - Reason for each item

The most important reason to maintain an item of clothing is that we wear it. That should be simple, right? Isn't that reason enough to save the bulk of our clothing? Not so quickly. The Pareto principle (or 80/20 rule) states that we wear 20% of our clothing 80% of the time. Uh-oh! That implies we don't wear the bulk of our clothes very often. We could reduce our wardrobes to one-fifth their original size and not miss a thing! As a result, we aim to distinguish our "favourite 20" from our "unworn 80"—that is, to find the pieces that fit, flatter, and suit our lifestyles.

A piece of clothing that suits you should be kept in your closet. In contrast, if an item does not fit, you cannot wear it; if you cannot, why retain it? Don't put yourself through the agony of keeping multiple clothing for different weights. If you maintain "fat clothing," you'll be depressed because you can't fit into them; if you keep "slim clothes," you'll be depressed because you can't fit into them. Instead, once you lose the weight, treat yourself to a new outfit. What a wonderful reason to skip dessert and go to the gym! Save only the clothing that fits you now, and go shopping for your new figure when it appears. (You're exempt if you're pregnant; but, if you haven't returned to your pre-baby weight by your child's first birthday, it's time to declutter.)

Items that compliment your figure are also acceptable in your closet. You'll avoid cluttering your wardrobe with "mistakes" if you learn which colours and shapes suit you best. Do you like to dress in fitting or flowing clothes? Pants with a pleat or plain fronts? Should you wear a little or a maxi skirt? Should you go for a crew or a v-neck? Choose the sleeve length that makes your arms seem sexier and the skirt length that best shows off your legs. Determine which colours look good with your skin tone and which ones bleach it out. Dress for your physique, not for trends: just because hip-huggers or cropped shirts are popular doesn't mean you should wear them. When choosing an outfit, consider if you'd be okay being photographed in it or running into your ex in it. If the answer is "no," it's out!

We also have excellent cause to preserve clothing that fits our lives and discard those that don't. List the tasks for which you need clothing, such as job, social occasions, gardening, house cleaning, and exercise, and then analyse your wardrobe appropriately. Resist the need to keep "fantasy" clothes; a wardrobe full of cocktail dresses and ball gowns will not turn you into a socialite. Instead, devote your space to what you'll wear "in real life." Consider whether a recent life change has changed your wardrobe requirements. For example, if you've quit your corporate job to work from home, you can get rid of your business suits; if you've relocated from Northumberland to Devon, you may get rid of your sheepskin coat.

Finally, consider a bad excuse to maintain an item of clothing: you paid "excellent money" for it. I know you feel guilty even thinking of throwing that cashmere sweater or those expensive heels —no matter how long you haven't worn them. You rationalise that if they're still in your closet, you haven't squandered your money (been there, done that!). There are two options for dealing with such clothing—and one of them is not to keep it. You may either sell the item and try to recuperate some of your money, or you can give it away and consider it a charity contribution.

In the latter instance, at the very least, the money "spent" will benefit a worthy cause!

E - Everything in its place

When arranging your clothes, keep in mind that your wardrobe is a separate zone. As a result, anything you wear should be confined within its furnishings, which might be a closet, dresser, armoire, or shelf unit. Keeping everything together helps you keep track of the size and contents of your wardrobe—and keeps you from rushing around half-naked hunting for your "lost" trousers! Allow your clothing to stray into other areas of the room or other rooms in the house: your sweaters should not be hanging over a chair, your socks should not be stacked in the corner, your shoes should not be reclining in the living room, and your shirts should not be hiding in your spouse's closet (at least not without permission).

Give everything a place within your wardrobe zone; it makes dressed in the morning so much easier. Set aside specific shelves for t-shirts, drawers for underwear, and parts of the wardrobe for jackets, suits, and dresses. If you've fully decluttered but still lack storage space, try several "space-saving" alternatives.

Sort your clothes into the Inner Circle, Outer Circle, and Deep Storage. This is where your "favourite 20%" should go. Devote your Inner Circle to the items you wear daily or weekly: socks, underwear, pyjamas, work clothing, weekend clothes, workout clothes, and everyday clothes. Keep these workhorses conveniently accessible in top drawers, middle shelves, and the centre area of your closet—not just to save time getting dressed but also to make them easy to put away. If returning them to their original locations is difficult, such as bending over, standing on a footstool, or moving a stack of objects, they will most likely end up on the floor, your bed, or a neighbouring chair.

Reserve your Outer Circle for clothes you only wear once or twice a month to once or twice a year. This category would most likely feature your dressier and formal apparel. Why retain them if you seldom ever wear them? Because chances are you'll be asked to a wedding, Christmas party, or other social occasions this year, and having something on hand is less stressful than having to go shopping. That doesn't imply you should have three tuxedos or five beautiful gowns on hand; only keep the bare necessities. Because such occasions are rare and far between, you can typically get away with wearing the same outfit again; unless you're a social diva, no one will remember (or care) what you wore to the last one.

Speciality and seasonal clothing, such as ski pants and beach suits, may also be found in your Outer Circle. Indeed, you may find it more practical to keep out-of-season clothing in your Outer Circle (for example, on the top shelf of your wardrobe or beneath the bed) and swap them with your Inner Circle at the right time of year. Heavy sweaters will be put away in the summer but accessible in the winter, while shorts and sundresses will be out of the way when it's chilly but accessible when it's nice. Take advantage of the chance to simplify as you go from one season to the next.

Deep Storage should include very little (if any) clothes. If you wish to preserve them, sentimental pieces (such as wedding, christening, and communion gowns) are possible choices. Deep Storage may also be used to save outgrown children's clothing for a younger sibling. Just be cautious where you keep them; attics, basements, and garages may be harsh conditions for fabric and may cause it to end up in the trash. Find a distant yet climate-controlled location inside the house if feasible.

A - All surfaces clear

Don't let items from your closets and dressers flow out onto the surfaces surrounding them; instead, make an effort to keep these areas clean. Hang everything up or put it in the hamper right away —don't drop it on the floor, plonk it on the bed, or pile it on a chair. Properly storing your clothing will keep them cleaner, minimise wrinkling, and make them simpler to find when you need them. At the very least, do it for the sake of your partner; no one wants to see someone else's dirty laundry scattered about! A "floordrobe" may rapidly detract from the atmosphere of a romantic evening or a quiet weekend morning.

Similarly, make every effort to keep the floor of your closet clear; a jumble of objects on the floor makes it easy for "intruders" to hide. Try to fit all of the items onto vertical Storage, such as shelves, shoe racks, closet rods, or hanging organisers. Modular systems are especially efficient and may be customised to meet your needs. This type of organising prevents clutter from accumulating and maintains your garments in excellent shape. The last thing you want to do when getting ready for a job interview or a first date is picking your blouse or jacket from the floor of your wardrobe.

Finally, if you have an armoire, avoid piling things on top of it. I realise it's tempting to utilise this high, out-of-the-way hiding area as a last-resort storage site. However, the surface is frequently neglected during housecleaning rounds, so whatever you store up there will quickly become dusty. Besides, dragging out a step stool every time you need to access anything is inconvenient. Worst case scenario, you may completely forget about the items up there. Keep it clean as you would any other surface in the house.

M - Modules

Consolidate your clothes, like your DVDs, office supplies, and culinary gadgets, into modules. The outcomes might be eye-opening! You may learn (much to your surprise) that you own ten pairs of black trousers, twenty white shirts, and thirty pairs of shoes. When you see them all together, you'll realise you have far more than enough. The goal is to keep them together, so you're never tempted to add to your collection. All of your skirts, pants, dresses, and jackets should be hung together. Keep pyjamas, gym clothing, and sweaters on separate shelves and socks and underwear in separate drawers. Be diligent about keeping things in order; if your yoga pants become friends with your work suits or your tank tops become friends with your tights, you never know what may happen!

You may further segment your "category" modules by colour, season, or kind if you like. In this case, you would keep all of your blue pants, brown jackets, and khaki shorts together. Similarly, you might categorise your shirts as sleeveless, short sleeve, or long sleeve, and your skirts as tiny, knee-length, or ankle-length. You may categorise your outfits as casual or formal and your suits as summer or winter weight. The more precise your modules, the easier it is to inventory what you have. You'll be able to see what you have too much of, what you have just enough of, and what you might still need, making it much easier to organise your wardrobe.

Do the same with accessories; just because they're little doesn't mean they should be overlooked. Consolidate your scarves and organise them by season. Consolidate your shoes and categorise them according to activity (how many pairs of sneakers do you have?). Consolidate your jewellery by categorising it as earrings, necklaces, brooches, rings, and bracelets. Consolidate your bags and categorise them according to colour, season, or purpose. Make a specific location for each category and ensure that its contents remain there. Accessories tend to roam and can find up in unexpected places, as anybody who has ever looked for a handbag or a set of earrings knows all too well.

When you've gathered everything, it's time to cull. If you find yourself with too many things in a single category (say, two dozen button-down shirts), keep just the best and most flattering—that's probably what you'll end up wearing anyway. Having a few extras is acceptable; few individuals can get by with only one shirt or pair of jeans. Even Buddhist monks are usually dressed in two robes! The issue arises when we have so many similar items that we rarely wear the majority of them. Excess is frequently the outcome of a quest for "perfection": the perfect pair of black slacks, the perfect white shirt, the perfect handbag. We keep purchasing and buying and buying till we have more than we need. Choose the greatest and most attractive parts of yourself, and then declutter the rest.

After you've consolidated and culled your goods, try to confine them as much as possible to keep them in order. This does not indicate that you should go out and buy twenty plastic containers. "Contain" can also imply "keep on a certain shelf, in a specific drawer, or a specific part of your closet." It might mean that all of your blue pants are on a multi-trouser hanger, all of your jeans are stacked together, or all of your ties are stored on a single rack. On the other hand, small goods should be stored in actual containers, such as trays, boxes, or baskets; for items such as pantyhose, scarves, watches, and jewellery, use trays, boxes, or baskets. It will keep things orderly and put a stop to their buildup.

L - Limits

Clothing is affordable and readily accessible in this era of mass manufacturing; we may pop down to our local mall and come back with a carload if we so choose. Furthermore, fashion is always changing; what is "in" one season is "out" the next, only to be replaced by a new set of must-have products. Our great-grandparents could only buy (and get) a few new outfits each year, but we have no such constraints. It's no surprise that our closets are overflowing!

That is why limitations are so essential in our minimalist wardrobes; they confine our clothing and accessories to a sensible size. We'd be buried beneath an avalanche of clothes if they weren't there! In the broadest sense, we should restrict our clothing to the amount of storage space available. If our armoires or drawers are overflowing, we need to stop the flow—and keep the contents from spilling into the room. Even if we can hold back the torrent, we don't want to teeter on the brink of disaster. The goal is not to cram our closets as full as possible but rather to eliminate enough items to provide some breathing room. When we have to wrestle our clothing out of the closet or crush them into drawers, it is not healthy for our clothes (or our stress levels). With that in mind, I'll amend my previous statement: we should restrict our wardrobe to no more than the amount of storage space available.

Set limitations on your nightwear, workout clothing, and "messy work" clothes (the worn-out stuff you reserve for gardening or painting). Depending on your washing and activity schedules, one to five clothes should be enough. Limit your accessories as well—scarves, ties, bags, and jewellery may quickly accumulate if we don't keep track of them. Calculate how many you wear in a normal week and establish a fair restriction; alternatively, limit them to the container in which they are stored.

Above all, have fun with your boundaries!

I - If one comes in, one goes out

We may purge and cleanse and purge—taking stuff to consignment stores, selling them on eBay, and donating them to charity—but our closets won't become any emptier until we stop the inflow. Our new purchases will undermine and impede our decluttering efforts. Fortunately, we may prevent this difficulty by adhering to the One In-One Out rule; if we offset each entering item with a departing one, we will not collect more than we currently have.

Fashion changes quicker than our clothes wear out, so if we buy new stuff every season, our wardrobes will rapidly become overcrowded. As a result, as we update our wardrobes, we must also cleanse them of the out-of-date, outgrown, and out-of-favour items. The easiest method to do this is to make a like-for-like trade: if you bring home a new pair of shoes, send an old pair packing; if you splurge on a new party dress, send an old one packing; and if you buy a new work suit, retire an old one. Then, rather than a stale record of styles past, your wardrobe will be a new, ever-changing collection.

When you were creating your modules, you may have noticed that you had too much in some categories and too little in others—for example, you may have enough pants to last a lifetime but very few skirts. This is a frequent problem since we tend to lean toward or stock up on particular goods when we find something we enjoy. In such a scenario, feel free to experiment with the One In-One Out rule to rebalance things. When you buy a new skirt, replace it with a pair of pants; do the same for any other categories that need to be adjusted. After you've rebalanced your clothing, you may resume swapping like-for-like.

Don't succumb to the temptation to cheat! You may be so eager to wear new clothing that decluttering an old one is the last thing on your thoughts on occasion. But guess what? If you don't do it right away, you won't be able to do it later. Use your eagerness to use your new clothes as a motivation to get rid of the old: don't take the tags off that new jacket until you've listed the old one on eBay or added it to your donation box. Make it a habit, and it will become second nature (and a lot simpler) over time. You're more likely to go shopping with a castoff in mind.

Finally, if your old clothes are "too excellent" to throw away, consider if you truly need anything new. What's the sense of expanding your wardrobe if your existing wardrobe serves its purpose? Don't feel obligated to follow fashion trends; they're nothing more than a marketing gimmick meant to take you from your money. Rather than purchasing each season's must-haves, invest in timeless classics. You'll have more money in your bank account, a larger closet, and a lot less decluttering to do.

N - Narrow it down

A minimalist wardrobe is essentially what is known as a "capsule wardrobe": a limited number of essential pieces that can be combined and matched to create a range of looks. The idea is intended to solve the problem of having "a wardrobe full of clothing and nothing to wear," and it entails selecting an intelligent colour, style, fabric, and accessory selections. Do you remember the Pareto principle? On the other hand, a capsule wardrobe is made up of the 20% of items you wear 80% of the time. You'll save money, free up closet space, and always appear well-dressed by limiting your wardrobe.

The goal is to choose a neutral colour, such as black, brown, grey, navy, cream, or khaki, and restrict foundation items (such as pants and skirts) to that shade.

In conclusion, your minimalist wardrobe should prioritise quality over quantity. Reduce your wardrobe to your most classic, adaptable, and well-made pieces, along with a few elegant accessories. You'll appear like a million bucks in a fraction of the time!

E - Everyday maintenance

Let us applaud ourselves for a job well done! We've made more room in our closets and learned to look great in less. Now, all we have to do is make sure things don't get out of hand again. We can keep our minimalist outfits at their new, simplified levels with a little daily upkeep.

First and foremost, resolve to keep your closet neat. When you remove an item of clothing, hang it, fold it, or otherwise store it in its correct location. By putting items in their proper modules, you'll always have a clear idea of what you own—and avoid the possibility of five new sweaters sneaking in unnoticed. Furthermore, if you adhere to the One In-One Out rule—swapping old things for new ones—you will never have to worry about your wardrobe increasing. As you continue to simplify, your closet will get more spacious.

Second, take good care of your clothes; since you don't have many of them, you can't afford to have a key piece ruined by a mud spatter or a frayed hem. Avoid wearing suede shoes in the rain or white trousers to your child's soccer game to minimise potential damage. A little preventative care goes a long way as well: repair little tears before they become large ones and remove stains before they become persistent. When you take care of your clothes, you won't need backups waiting in the wings.

Third, avoid shopping malls. Don't shop for the sake of enjoyment, amusement, or boredom; that's when you get into trouble! You've worked hard to get rid of the excess in your wardrobe, but one shopping trip might put you back in the same situation. You know the scenario: you're browsing around a department shop when a lovely outfit catches your attention. After 45 minutes, you're going out the door with it—along with matching shoes, a handbag, a wrap, earrings, and a few other things you found along the way. To prevent temptation, don't enter a store (or browse a retailer's website) unless you truly need something. Establish a wardrobe inventory and bring it with you when you go shopping; if you have twenty-three shirts on your list, you're far less likely to buy a twenty-fourth.

Finally, declutter with the change of seasons. Fall and spring are excellent seasons to rethink your wardrobe. Take some time to browse over your jackets and sweaters before bringing them out for the winter. Our tastes evolve, as do our bodies, and so does fashion. That jacket you adored last year may now appear old, obsolete, or unattractive to you, and those slim pants may have gotten a little too narrow since you last wore them. Perhaps that cashmere sweater has a moth hole, or that "it" thing you purchased is suddenly hopelessly "out." Get rid of everything you don't believe you'll wear, and start the new season with more closet space!

Dining Room And Kitchen

Many of us would select the kitchen as the most practical area in the house if asked. After all, it is where we store, prepare, serve, and eat the food that keeps us alive. It is also a popular spot for family gatherings. Given its importance in our lives, it's no surprise that the kitchen has many things! Too many things, on the other hand, might reduce the room's functionality and make it unpleasant to work and hang out in. So let's see how we can simplify things and make this place as efficient as possible.

S - Start over

Have you ever strolled into a kitchen showroom (or perused the pages of your favourite designer magazine) and dreamed about trading in your current kitchen for the one on display? Did you feel envious of its glistening surfaces, imagining how great it would be to cook in such a sleek and practical environment? Have you ever believed that if you only had more cabinet storage, your life would be perfect?

Most of the time, what draws us to showroom kitchens isn't the high-end equipment, specialised granite, or beautiful cabinetry—it's space! Display kitchens are typically clean, minimalist, and devoid of clutter, with only a few appliances and tableware. That is what makes them so beautiful and welcoming. The good news is that you don't have to spend a fortune on renovations to have this appearance. Simply decluttering your kitchen may give it a dramatic change.

Remember how we talked about moving day and how great it felt to unpack your belongings into a clean, uncluttered space? Remember how pleasant it was to line up your plates, glasses, utensils, and gadgets in perfect order on those lovely empty shelves and cabinets? Unfortunately, things have likely grown a little more busy and disorganised between then and now. Don't worry; we'll replicate that first day by Starting Over, one cabinet at a time.

To accomplish this, empty each drawer, cabinet, cupboard, and shelf in turn. As usual, don't be tempted to leave anything because you "know" you'll put it back. That is unethical! Remove everything from the kitchen, including plates, coffee cups, glasses, forks, spoons, knives, pots, pans, gadgets, appliances, food, foil, takeout containers, and even the contents of your "trash" drawer. Remember, the goal isn't to choose and choose what we'll get rid of, but to pick and select what we'll keep. After you've taken everything out, you'll meticulously inspect it all and restore only your best, most helpful, and most important objects to their proper places. Pretend you're furnishing a brand-new dream kitchen, similar to the ones seen in magazines; why should yours be any less spectacular?

If you have any worries about thoroughly emptying the cabinets, this approach comes with a wonderful bonus: the fantastic chance to clean those cabinets. How long has it been since they've been scrubbed? Kitchens become oily and dirty throughout the cooking process, and while we're quite good at keeping the surfaces clean, we often forget about the insides of our cabinets. Grime, dust, and spills accumulate over time and create unsanitary conditions. So, while you're getting rid of the clutter, get rid of the dirt as well (see how efficient we minimalists are!). Scrub them clean, and you'll have a "new" start!

T - Transfer, Treasure, or Trash?

While cleaning out your cabinets, cupboards, and counters, you're bound to stumble find a few items for your Trash pile. If you haven't emptied your pantry in a while, most of it may be food; check the expiration dates on everything you touch, and toss anything rotten, expired, or otherwise beyond its prime. Spices, sauces, and condiments all have a short shelf life, so don't overlook them while decluttering. If that bottle of soy sauce is older than your kid's, discard it and replace it as required. Do the same with other perishables, especially if you can't remember how long you've had them or when you last used them.

Other trash, such as chipped dishes, cracked glasses, and twisted or mangled silverware, may also be hiding in your kitchen (like the fork that got caught in the garbage disposal). Give your meal the attention it deserves by serving it on (and with) immaculate tableware. Don't keep these damaged parts as backups for your more valuable items; they're difficult to repair, depressing to look at, and unsafe to use. Send them to the sky's Great Kitchen Table! Discard damaged devices and appliances as well; if you haven't already taken the effort to fix them, you don't need them.

All goods that are beneficial to someone other than you go in your Transfer pile. For some reason, we tend to amass far more cookware than we require or use daily. Some of it finds its way into our lives as wedding and housewarming presents, while others come as spontaneous purchases. Some goods may have looked useful when we bought them, but they turned out to be too difficult or time-consuming for our lives; thus, donate that pasta machine or ice cream maker to someone who would appreciate it. As you go through your belongings, be honest with yourself; if you avoid using your food processor because it's difficult to clean, now is the time to let it go.

Don't forget that food may also go into your Transfer pile. Our tastes and dietary demands vary over time, and certain items' shelf life might outlast our desire for them. We may become bored of tomato soup before we finish it or decide that fresh fruit is preferable to canned fruit on our shelves. Don't feel terrible; instead, see it as a fantastic opportunity to do a nice act! Donate any unused canned or packaged goods to a food bank or soup kitchen in your community. Your pantry scraps can help someone else avoid going hungry.

You could find it tough to get rid of some kitchen things because you're afraid you'll need them someday (and you're quite sure it'll be the day after you get rid of them). If this is the case, add a box labelled Temporarily Undecided. Put items in it that you don't use daily but believe you might need soon, such as the bread machine, muffin tins, and fancy cake decorating tools. Mark the box with a date and donate whatever you don't retrieve after a certain amount of time (say six months or a year). It's a fantastic method to deal with goods that are "on the fence"; they're available if needed but won't take up valuable space in your cabinets and drawers. Better still, you'll get a taste of what life is like without them—and you could discover that you don't miss them at all.

Your Treasure pile should only contain items that you rely on, appreciate, or utilise daily. These contenders are competing for a coveted position in your cupboards and must demonstrate their worth. We'll study them attentively as we go through the stages below to determine what deserves a spot in our kitchens.

R - Reason for each item

The kitchen is an excellent area to converse with your belongings. Some objects have been hiding in the shadows for so long that you may no longer recognise them. This is your time to reconnect and ensure that your relationship is still mutually beneficial.

What exactly are you, and what do you do? We shouldn't have to ask, but let's face it: we don't always know what we're looking for. There's a kitchen gadget for every possible activity these days, and just because that pineapple corer or pastry wheel seemed necessary when we purchased it doesn't guarantee we'll remember it in a few years. A little uncertainty is not a good thing in this instance. If you don't know what anything does, it's probably not necessary in your kitchen. Send it on—it may make a great present for a culinary friend who might know what to do with it.

How frequently do I use you? The million-dollar question! Items that get the response "every day" or "once a week" may begin to reappear in your cabinets. However, just because you only use the turkey baster once a year does not mean you have to get rid of it; such knowledge may merely assist you in deciding where to keep it. If you use anything less than once a year, you should consider whether it's worth the space it's taking up. It's extremely improbable that you'll miss it nine times out of 10.

Do you have a twin? Kitchen goods, like office supplies, appear to increase on their own. You cannot use more than one potato peeler or can opener simultaneously unless you are exceptionally skilled. Furthermore, if one fails, you can quickly replace it. Get rid of the doubles to make room for something more valuable.

Are you too good to be put to use? I'm sure your equipment didn't see this one coming! Wedding china and inherited silverware may get fairly cocky, thinking they can sit about for decades doing nothing. They're often correct: they're hidden away in dining hutches and barely see the light of day. We're too attached to them to get rid of them, and we're too afraid to utilise them (lest we break a piece and have to hunt for a replacement). In the case of silver, we could just fear polishing them. Here's an unconventional idea: instead of the entire service, maintain simply one or two place settings for décor or romantic candlelight dinners with your partner.

E - Everything in its place

Because the kitchen serves various tasks, from food preparation to eating to bill payment, separating it into activity zones can help us stay organised and efficient. Determine the locations where you will conduct certain duties, such as preparing, cooking, serving, eating, washing up, and trash disposal, and keep associated tools and equipment in their allocated zones. Keep the knives where you cut, the pots near the stove, and the dishwashing solutions beneath the sink, for example. To keep pens, chequebooks, and calculators from stacking up on the counter or making their way into your spice cabinet, assign distinct locations to incidental chores such as bill-paying.

Reserve a specific location within your zones for every last thing; it's the greatest method to keep order in such a busy environment. The dishes should always be perfectly placed, and the cups and glasses should fall into position like a chorus line. Forks, knives, spoons, pots, pans, and appliances should all have particular locations to which they should return. Consider drawing imaginary lines around each object as if it were an allocated parking place. Stick small sticky labels ("pasta pot," "saucepan," "cereal bowls") to remind you (and family members) where everything goes. Otherwise, you may wind up with a chaotic jumble—the ideal habitat for junk to hide.

At the same time, allocate objects to your Inner Circle, Outer Circle, and Deep Storage. Your Inner Circle should include the plates, pots, pans, cutlery, drinkware, gadgets, appliances, and meals you use regularly. They should be within arm's reach, in the zone where they're usually needed; you shouldn't have to climb a stepladder to get your coffee mug or cross the room to get your paring knife. Dedicate your most easily accessible storage areas to these goods, and keep them clear of other, infrequently used objects. That way, you won't have to go through a drawer full of other items to find your measuring spoons. Such organisation makes the task of preparing and presenting a meal much more enjoyable!

Store goods in your Outer Circle that you use less than once a week but more than once a year. Cake pans, cookie sheets, muffin tins, waffle irons, blenders, salad spinners, ice cream makers, bread machines, crock pots, and champagne glasses are common items. Reserve your upper cabinets, lower drawers, and deeper nooks for these less often used items; you may need to bend, stretch, or reach a bit to grab them. They shouldn't be too difficult to find, but they don't have to be right at your fingers.

Finally, place the kitchen and dining goods you only use once a year (or less) into Deep Storage. Turkey roasters, punch bowls, gravy boats, soufflé dishes, dessert stands, serving platters, and specialised linens—basically, items you exclusively use for holidays or entertaining—are probable contenders for this category. Place these in the highest, lowest, and farthest reaches of your kitchen or dining area. If you don't have the room, you may store them in the garage, basement, or attic; just be certain to adequately wrap or enclose them to keep out dirt, moisture, and roaming creatures. However, just because you can place items in Deep Storage doesn't imply you have to. If you don't need such goods for entertaining (or can borrow them if necessary), don't keep them at all.

A - All surfaces clear

Our kitchen countertops are highly significant surfaces since they are utilised for food preparation three times each day (or more, if we count those mid-afternoon munchies and late-night snacks). It's virtually difficult to cook a beautiful dinner when they're cluttered with kitchen gadgets, filthy dishes, knickknacks, mail, or recipe books. And if you don't have room to wash, cut, slice, dice, pare, and peel, you're more inclined to microwave frozen food or order takeout. Don't let clutter keep you from enjoying a nutritious, home-cooked meal!

Cooking is tough when you're continuously shifting items out of the way or are restricted to a small piece of the countertop. As a result, your kitchen surfaces should only include products that you use regularly (if that). Consider wall-mounted racks for spices, knives, and other utensils, as well as hanging baskets for fruits and vegetables to keep them off the countertops. Microwaves, toaster ovens, and coffee machines that attach under top cabinets can help save room. Skip the cutesy trinkets and cookie jars for a more appealing and practical kitchen, and instead go for sleek and minimalist. I assure you that merely clearing the clutter from your counters will revitalise you and encourage you to create some culinary magic.

The kitchen has long been considered the heart of the home, a place for families to meet and spend quality time together; but, since it is such a busy place, its countertops are magnets for clutter. Make sure that anybody who drops a toy, book, newspaper, or piece of mail takes it with them when they leave the room. (Or tell them that it could be in your next dish!) Keep an eye on the floor as well, and keep it clear of book bags, toys, and pet supplies; while moving large pots and boiling liquids, anything underfoot can be a formula for catastrophe. Make a thorough scan of the space, returning all stray things to their proper placements.

Similarly, keep your kitchen and dining tables tidy and ready for the next meal. Such surfaces are utilised for a range of activities in most families, which is to be expected. (Variety is a wonderful thing!) However, don't let homework assignments, craft projects, or tax returns consume these tables, leaving them worthless for their intended function. I've seen dining tables transformed into sponta-neous storage units piled high with papers, books, magazines, toys, art equipment, and other odd items. This surface is undoubtedly useful for flex space, but the dining table should contain no more than the next meal's accessories when not in use. If you seldom use the dining room for eating, try removing the table and repurposing the space (like a home office).

After you've finished cooking:

- Put all of the equipment and ingredients away and wash down the surface.
- After each meal, clear the table and wash pots, pans, and dirty dishes (or at least load them into the dishwasher).
- Scan your kitchen surfaces before going to bed every night and tuck any stray objects away. Finally, don't consider a dinner "finished" until every surface has been cleared.

It's a joy to wake up the next day with a clean countertop and an empty sink!

M - Modules

You've probably gotten a good start on this stage because the idea of the module comes easily in the kitchen. If you already keep your cutlery, spices, and cake decorating tools together, you're well on your way to a more organised area.

Consolidating like with like is especially useful in the kitchen, where duplicate supplies and surplus components are prevalent. It allows you to cut down on the essentials and stops you from purchasing unneeded extras because you can see at a glance what you already have. If you store all of your baking supplies in one drawer, you'll be less inclined to buy a second bottle of vanilla because you can't locate the first. If you know you have six coffee cups, you'll think twice before buying a souvenir mug on your next vacation. If you can see how many forks, spoons, and knives you have, you may refuse grandma's flatware and give it to your sister instead.

Modules illustrate how some objects have collected (often undetected) over time. They force us to ponder questions such as, "Why do we have eighteen drinking cups for our family of four?" "Will we ever utilise twenty pairs of chopsticks?" and "Why do I need two meat thermometers, three corkscrews, and four cinnamon jars?" Duplicates are a fantastic way to declutter. It's quick and simple since we don't have to stress over options or worry about doing "without" something (we'll still have one, after all). It also frees up space in our cabinets and drawers, making it considerably easier to get our hands on something when we need it. When we're cooking, the ability to swiftly identify a certain ingredient or utensil might be the difference between "wonderful" and "disaster!"

Gather your food into modules as well:

- Put cereals, soups, and canned goods in designated parts on your shelves.
- Keep cheese, veggies, and condiments in their portions of the refrigerator.
- Organise cans and bottles of beverages by kind.

Organising your provisions in this manner minimises overbuying and waste because you can rapidly examine your inventory before heading to the store. You could even realise that you have more of something than you'll ever need; rather than letting it go to waste, give the extra to a food bank. On the other hand, you'll know where you need to stock up and can prevent running out unexpectedly.

Whether we like it or not, most of our kitchens have a "junk" drawer where we keep ketchup packets, takeout menus, batteries, birthday candles, twist ties, tea lights, sewing needles, scissors, plastic cutlery, and other strange objects that are too tiny, few, or uncategorisable to fit anyplace else. Is it OK to have such a mishmash of items in a minimalist kitchen? Sure, but only if the following criteria are met: Examine every item, keeping just those you'll truly need, and putting them all in a single "utility" module (same drawer, the new and improved name!). Put comparable things in ziplock bags or drawer organiser slots. There is no need to classify anything as "junk" if it is freely accessible, simply recognisable, and really helpful.

L - Limits

Limiting our culinary items maintains them under control—and our kitchens appearing like the clean, tranquil environments we admire in magazines.

Let's start with tableware because most of us have considerably more than we need. Consider restricting your plates, cups, bowls, glasses, and utensils to the size of your family; if you only have four people in your home, why clutter your cupboards with sixteen place settings? Extra dinnerware only serves as an excuse to postpone dishwashing, making the task more difficult and unpleasant when we do eventually get around to it.

But, you say, what about the guests? By all means, keep your entertainment habits in mind while you go through your supplies. Determine the most people you typically host and preserve extra dinnerware to fit the gathering. The crucial term here is "frequently," instead of once every three years or so when you host a holiday dinner. If you're planning a large event, you can always borrow items from family and friends; most will have extras they're happy to offer. If you must retain all of your place settings, keep only the ones you use daily in your cabinets, and store the remainder in Deep Storage until they are needed.

We'd also be wise to keep our appliances and devices to a minimum. Just because there is a gadget for every culinary activity does not imply that we must own it. Keep the ones you use the most frequently, and get rid of the others. Do the same thing with all of those plastic takeaway containers. They rapidly pile up since we hate to throw away such potentially valuable objects; yet, they frequently end up in a tangled mess, cluttering up our cupboards. Determine the amount you require, select the most durable and flexible parts, then recycle or give the surplus.

Keep the décor in your kitchen to a minimum. A single bowl of fresh fruit or flowers is far more beautiful than a counter piled high with trinkets. Instead of ornamental items, use culinary products to freshen up the space:

- Pasta and beans look beautiful in glass jars.
- Spices are pleasant to the sight as well as the flavour.
- Sprigs of lavender or other herbs give your kitchen a charming, natural aspect.

Appliances may be both attractive and functional: a toaster, blender, or coffee maker in a bright colour or sleek form may be all you need to brighten up your kitchen. Most essential, keep the number of objects per surface to a minimum so that you can cook a meal without putting things away.

Furthermore, if space is limited, keep the amount of food you store to a minimum. Keep enough for an emergency, but consider whether you truly need a year's supply of beans, rice, coffee, or canned foods. Make an effort to "eat through your pantry" regularly and restock it with new goods so that food does not spoil or go to waste. To avoid buying (and keeping) excessive amounts, keep track of your inventory and prepare shopping lists before heading to the grocery store.

Finally, think about utilising limitations to clear out the clutter in your diet. Obesity and health issues can be caused by an excess of food or specific components, such as salt, fat, sugar, and preservatives. Limiting your diet to basic, nutritious meals (such as fresh fruits and vegetables) helps you avoid the harmful impacts of highly processed foods. The benefits are twofold: by limiting the snacks and sweets in your cupboards, you will simplify both your figure and your kitchen! Limits are a wonderful alternative to going cold turkey when making a dietary adjustment. If you want to eat less meat, limit yourself to once or twice a week; if you want to drink less alcohol, limit yourself to one glass of wine instead of two; and if you need to cut back on pastries, do so just once a week (or monthly) as a special treat. You may live a healthy lifestyle without feeling deprived in this way.

I - If one comes in, one goes out

Purge a comparable item every time you bring a new one into the kitchen from now on. As a result, you'll never have as many cups, plates, forks, spoons, or garlic presses as you have now. When we obtain a new set of dishes, we often forget to get rid of the old ones. The issue is that the old items are fully functional most of the time—we simply replace them because our tastes have changed or we want a new appearance. So the old set is stowed away in the depths of our cabinets, "just in case" we need any extras. Alternatively, we may inherit newcomers or receive them as presents, and even if we don't like them, we may feel compelled to provide them with a home. Whatever the case may be, our cupboards become overflowing with an unusual mixture of plates, glasses, cutlery, and service ware. No more! We will no longer keep every plate or cup that comes our way from now on. We'll reduce down to our most recent, greatest, or most attractive specimens, and we'll get rid of the old to create room for the new.

A similar issue arises with kitchen equipment. It's difficult to throw out an old piece, especially if we've replaced it before its time has come. As a result, ancient toasters, coffee makers, crock pots, and grills find refuge in the darkest depths of our cupboards. On the other hand, such appliances are heavy and hard to store, and getting rid of them may free up a lot of room. Instead of sheltering these retirees, donate them to someone in need—a college student or young couple may be overjoyed to get such essential things. Donations will also be appreciated by charity stores, charities, and homeless shelters.

Apply the One In-One Out rule to foods, especially those used slowly and over time, such as spices, seasonings, sauces, and condiments. Such goods tend to stay in our drawers and refrigerator shelves long past their expiration date; we buy them for a certain meal, stash them away, and then entirely forget about them. Then, the next time we need one, we go to the shop and buy a new one. If you happen to have a spare bottle of soy sauce, chilli powder, or maple syrup, don't keep it; instead, replace it with the new item. Your shelves will be less cluttered, and your food will taste much better.

Finally, let's talk about cookbooks and recipes—many more

appear to enter the house than leave it. They grow slowly over time, and we seldom replace old ones; instead, we simply add to our collection. Recipes, in particular, seem to accumulate, flowing into our lives from all angles: magazines, family, friends, neighbours, and the Internet. We'll have more recipes than days in the year to prepare before we realise it! Rather than archiving them all, keep your selection current; if you find a better guidebook for a certain cuisine or a better recipe for a particular meal, discard the old one. Consider your collection to be dynamic rather than static; allow it to grow to fit your changing likes and diet.

N - Narrow it down

Therefore, it is up to you to establish your own "enough" and narrow down your culinary arsenal appropriately. Choosing multi-functional products over single-use items is a particularly effective strategy. Cherry pitters, melon ballers, bagel slicers, pizzelle irons, lobster shears, strawberry hullers, and crepe makers don't generally justify the space they take up in your kitchen cabinets unless you use them frequently. Instead, choose basic implementations that can handle a range of tasks. Similarly, having a whole set of skillets and saucepans isn't always essential; one or two in popular sizes is usually adequate.

Similarly, avoid amassing dinnerware in unusual sizes and forms (such as egg cups and sushi plates) favour adaptable, all-purpose dishes. Rather than storing both "good" and "everyday" china, select just one set and utilise it for all occasions. Reduce your glasses as well. You don't need a distinct vessel for each beverage if you don't own a restaurant, such as wine glasses, champagne glasses, whiskey glasses, beer glasses, martini glasses, water glasses, and juice glasses.

Consider getting rid of the expensive specialist equipment as well. Going out to dine can be more enjoyable than setting up, running, and cleaning a complicated gadget. Instead of dragging out a cappuccino machine, spend a wonderful afternoon at the coffee shop; instead of bothering with an ice cream maker, take the family to the ice cream parlour; and instead of hoarding bakeware, head to the patisserie when you have a sweet craving. Similarly, if you don't prepare anything difficult, you don't need professional appliances with all the bells and whistles. Take pleasure in the challenge of making meals with few tools; it's a focused, meditative, and rewarding way to cook.

When simplifying your kitchen, remember that the incredible diversity of cooking in certain cultures is done with the most basic of pots and utensils. Delicious, gratifying meals are created by our imagination in the kitchen, not by the equipment in our cupboards. Good food does not come from expensive plates and fussy serving ware; it comes from the hands and the heart and can be eaten in one simple bowl, as any Buddhist monk will tell you.

E - Everyday maintenance

Because the kitchen is such a hub of activity, it requires daily upkeep and all-day maintenance!

Things can quickly spin out of hand here if we don't keep an eye on things. Dirty dishes, pots, and pans accumulate in the sink; food, gadgets, and packaging accumulate on the counter; bills, homework, and newspapers accumulate on the table; toys, backpacks, and grocery bags accumulate on the floor; and leftovers accumulate in the refrigerator. In general, the more people in your family, the more things wind up in the kitchen. Eventually, the clutter will grow so overpowering that you won't be able to cook (or enjoy) a meal there.

When you're done cooking, put away all of your devices, utensils, and ingredients. After you've finished eating, clean up any leftover food or tools on the table and counters. After using the dishes, immediately wash them or load them into the dishwasher. It is preferable to spend a few minutes cleaning up after each meal rather than confronting the chore when preparing the next; a stack of dirty dishes may rapidly damper your motivation to prepare. Observe this rule: never leave the kitchen with dishes in the sink. Simply wipe the slate clean after each meal to avoid this. (At a bare minimum, never go to bed with dishes in the sink.) It's great to have a fresh start every day, but it's even better to have one at each meal!

Furthermore, keep an eye out for OPC (other people's clutter) in the kitchen. Your kitchen table, counters, or breakfast bar are almost certainly in regular use if you have a family. Books, toys, games, mail, and papers will all make their way there, and they won't always depart on their own (i.e., with the person who brought them in). Assure that all home members realise that the kitchen surfaces are flex space and should be thoroughly cleaned after usage. If that doesn't work, backfire wayward objects back to their rightful owners as quickly as possible. Remember that clutter breeds clutter; your teenager is more likely to leave a magazine or a bag of chips on a cluttered table than on a clean one.

Finally, the kitchen is an excellent location for a Once-A-Day Declutter. Something can always go in this room, whether it's yesterday's newspaper or last week's leftovers. Make it a practice to frequently inspect your refrigerator, freezer, and pantry shelves for expired or outdated foods (or those you don't want to consume) and dispose of them. Commit to getting rid of at least one thing every day, whether it's spoiled food, an extra coffee mug, an orphaned utensil, a mismatched plate, or a seldom-used device. You could probably survive for a year on the contents of your junk drawer alone. Consider this: your cupboards will become roomier with each passing day!

6

Your Finances

EVERYONE ENJOYS A GOOD DEAL, and retailers are well aware of this. To remain competitive, they are always devising new and inventive ways to encourage people to visit their businesses, such as newspaper coupons, special promotions, frequent-buyer discounts, and so on.

The actual benefit for you is that you no longer have to pay full price for anything unless you want to. With a little research, planning, and organisation, you can obtain excellent bargains on a variety of personal and home products. The advice in this chapter will assist you in maximising the purchasing power of your cash. Whatever your budget, you can obtain what you desire at a reasonable price. The best part is that you can accomplish it without a lot of headaches and bother.

Pay Off Your Debts

Your grandparents, like mine, are possibly survivors of the Second World War. My grandparents had one unbreakable rule regarding money: if they didn't have the cash in hand, they didn't buy things. They had never had a debt throughout their life, except the mortgage on their home. They simply refused to participate in the post–World War II purchase now–pay later attitude that has turned us into a country of debtors and consumers. When they required new furniture or a big item, they used money from their "contingency" fund, or if the fund was empty, they waited until they had saved enough money by saving a little each month.

Many people from our parents' and our parents' parents' generations were raised in this manner. Given that debt is one of the major sources of emotional and psychological stress in our lives, many of us would benefit by living in this way today.

If you are one of the many millions of people in the UK who have a credit card or instalment debt, there are a few things you can do:

1. You can take steps to get out of debt on your own.

This is sitting down and calculating exactly how much you owe, then creating a strategy to pay it off as swiftly and systematically as possible, even if it may take many years. It also entails establishing a commitment to yourself to avoid debt in the future. This method is feasible, but it takes discipline, dedication, and a thorough commitment to overcoming the stress created by debt.

2. If you believe you are in over your head and are beginning to believe you will never be able to get out on your own, you can seek assistance.

Live On Half Of Your Earnings And Save The Other Half

It is believed that less than 10% of people in the UK are fortunate to have all of their current and future financial requirements met. Many persons who will retire in the next twenty-five years will be able to live on little more than their pension. And few individuals are wagering money that their pensions will be an adequate or even a viable source of retirement income in the coming years.

We have evolved into a country of spenders rather than savers. While it is true that many individuals have been forced to live above their means as a result of rising living costs and a fall in the value of the pound, it is also true that we spend far more than we need to on things we don't need.

94

Take a careful look at how you spend your money if you're feeling so out of control with your spending that you believe you won't be able to save a large percentage of your salary. If you believe you won't be able to make significant savings in your spending, start by reducing your spending by simply 10% or 15% over the following year. The next year, reduce your spending by another 10 to 15%, ultimately up to 50%.

Almost 80% of the items in this book will help you save money. Living simply does not entail living cheaply or feeling deprived. On the contrary, it is an opportunity to reconnect with what is truly essential in your life and achieve a level of moderation that will provide you with a sense of satisfaction and stability and a sense of control.

If you've been living on the edge, reaching the point where you can set aside a significant percentage of your monthly income to cover your future requirements can put you back in control and go a long way toward simplifying your life.

Change Your Shopping Habits

If you have problems resisting the temptation to spend, make it difficult for yourself by going shopping but leaving your cash, chequebook, and credit cards at home.

For many people, purchasing is only a habit. Any habit may be broken by substituting another activity for the problematic one. Make a list of things you can do instead of shopping so that the next time you are tempted to spend money on items you don't need, you'll have something else to do.

Take a stroll, meet up with a friend, go to the library, or take a cold shower, for example, to avoid wasting time shopping. Though you may initially feel starved by the lack of shopping in your life, there is ultimately amazing freedom in not having to buy.

Make use of the Buddy System. If you've determined you really must have something, bring a buddy who is familiar with your purchasing patterns and sympathetic to your wish to change them. Have a buddy monitor your purchases to ensure that you only buy the item you intended to buy. But make sure you choose the appropriate pal.

Pay for everything with a debit card. This makes it a little more difficult than paying with cash or a credit card.

Examine advertisements with a jaundiced eye. The "thrill" of purchasing is addicting. You have to do it again once the adrenaline has worn off. That is what advertising relies on. It is much simpler to keep your money if you are aware of the power advertising has on it.

Minimise Your Needs Of Goods And Services

One of the eighties' myths was that the more goods we had and the more help we hired, the easier our lives would become. In the process of simplifying, I discovered the exact opposite is true.

Rethinking your purchasing patterns and changing the way you shop will help you eliminate the "goods" that are taking up space in your life. Many of the other steps outlined in this book will help you reduce your reliance on "services."

For example, once you begin simplifying, your house will be so simple to maintain that you won't need a cleaning lady; your meals will be so simple that you won't need a cook; your errands will be so organised that you won't need a chauffeur; your wardrobe will be so minimal that you won't need a fashion consultant; your investments will be consolidated so you won't need a bookkeeper, and your purchases will be limited your phone system is so direct that you won't require an answering service; Your lawn will be eliminated, eliminating the need for a gardener; your home will be decluttered, eliminating the need for a professional organiser; your relationships will be cleaned up, eliminating the need for a psychotherapist; and your health and fitness program will be so simple that you will not require a personal trainer.

Just scheduling (not to mention rescheduling), arranging for transportation, getting people to do things correctly, arranging to pay them, and finding someone to take their place when they quit (which they don't do until about the time you've trained them) is complicated enough for me to avoid most of these "services" like the plague.

Again, this is a matter of personal preference. We must individually determine when the products and services in our lives cease to make our lives simpler and begin to become a burden. Our objective was to structure our lives to easily take care of most of our wants and belongings on our own. We've given ourselves a whole new sense of independence by removing most of the things and services we believed we couldn't live without.

Pay Off Your Mortgage

If you're living in your dream home, intend to stay there, and your mortgage payments are within your means, you might want to consider taking steps to pay off your mortgage early. Alternatively, you may pay it off altogether.

For years, we've been told that the tax benefits of house ownership make it advantageous to carry a mortgage. You'll need to examine your situation and maybe check with an accountant, but the savings aren't all that big when the facts are calculated. Furthermore, many people realise that the independence of owning their house altogether much surpasses any tax advantages.

There are various approaches to mortgage payoffs:

1. Lump sum payments. If you receive large cash infusions on top of your regular salary, consider using them to pay down your mortgage. However, before making a large payment, ensure that your lender will re-calculate your loan and reduce your monthly payments.

2. Additional principal payments. By making the next month's principal payment along with your regular monthly payment, you can significantly reduce the term of your mortgage and save thousands of pounds over the life of your loan. Your lender will need to provide you with a copy of the amortisation schedule. Alternatively, if you have a variable rate loan, your lender will provide you with the calculation to determine the next month's principal payment at no cost.

3. Because the payment amount applied to the principal grows

with each payment; there may come a time when the increased principal payment becomes too much for you to handle. If this occurs, you can simply pay whatever amount you find comfortable toward the principal each month. You'll still save a lot of money on interest payments and be able to pay off your mortgage faster than you would have otherwise.

4. Sell your home and move to a smaller, lower-cost residence. Depending on the amount of equity you have in your home and the real estate values in the area where you now live and where you would be moving to, you may be able to use the proceeds from the sale of your current home to pay for your new home in full or significantly reduce the amount of the new mortgage. Again, you should consult with your accountant.

Any of these mortgage payoff plans presume that you have paid off any other outstanding obligations, such as credit cards or instalment loans, and that you have enough money set aside for emergencies and investments. Paying off your home early will not necessarily make your life easier right away, but it will free you out of the perpetual psychological strain of monthly mortgage payments.

Buy A Used Car The Next Time You Need One

When you consider that a new automobile loses 30% or more of its value the instant you drive it off the forecourt, you have to ask why anyone would ever buy a new car.

A large proportion of new-car customers swap in their vehicles every two to three years. These trade-ins are a great way to get a good deal on a used automobile. They've often been carefully driven and well maintained, so it's very simple to pay a technician to assess whether there are any serious flaws. In general, if an automobile develops issues, it will do so within the first ten to fifteen thousand kilometres.

Also, keep in mind that after two years, the value of a car has dropped by another 30% from its original price. So, if you buy directly from the owner rather than a used car dealer, you can save up to 60% off the car's original sticker price.

Not only will buying a used car save you money and, hopefully, the hassle of financing and monthly payments, but if you buy care-fully, you'll have a car that has already had the bugs worked out of it, and you can probably count on it for many thousands of miles of trouble-free driving.

Teach Your Children Financial Responsibility

We all want the best for our children, and it can be difficult to say no at times. But I can't help but wonder what kind of lessons we're teaching our children when we spend money on glitz and glitter "image builders," especially when we can't afford them.

As we develop new spending habits for ourselves, whether out of desire, necessity, or both, we should also develop sensible purchasing habits for our children. Children are flexible and may learn to live within appropriate boundaries. We just need to make sure they understand what the boundaries are. Teach your children to save half of their allowance or part-time earnings. Kids, like us, may learn that we don't have to have everything we see or everything the Joneses have. Kids, like us, can learn that there are alternatives: if they get the gold trim on the car, they can't have the new dirt bike. Children can learn to budget so that their costs do not exceed their income. Children can learn how advertisers appeal to our emotions rather than our needs, just as we do. Children can learn that if they don't have the money, they can't afford it and that buying on credit can lead to serious financial problems.

One of the most powerful gifts we can give our children is the ability to manage their money. Not only will it ultimately simplify their lives, but it will also simplify ours.

7

Your Work

ALBERT EINSTEIN, the great physicist who gave the world the theory of relativity, also pondered more commonplace topics like labour. He previously described his working habits in three simple guidelines.

Out of clutter, find simplicity.
From discord, find harmony.
In the middle of difficulty lies opportunity.

This wisdom is more relevant today than ever before, as working men and women struggle to maintain a sense of order and control in their fast-paced, technology-driven professional lives. Working effectively has become a science in and of itself. The good news is that there are several methods to simplify your workplace and office space. We'll go through some essential ideas here.

Pro-Knowledged Secrets

Working in these ultra-competitive times is unquestionably difficult. It certainly keeps you guessing. You can achieve virtually anything if you keep calm and organised.

First and foremost -

When many tasks competing for your attention, you must decide what gets done first. The strategies listed below can assist you in prioritising and planning your workload.

Understand what's important. According to Peter F Drucker, PhD author of Managing for Results, many business situations follow the 80/20 rule. For example, if you make 80 per cent of your sales to 20 per cent of your clients or utilise 80 per cent of your material from 20 per cent of your files. Prioritise the 20%—those individuals or tasks that can help you achieve your goals—and let the rest go.

When required, prevent flames. Your day might start great, only to be derailed by "emergencies" by lunchtime. Take action when a crisis occurs, but don't exaggerate the situation. It may be very urgent, or it could simply be essential. Learn to tell the difference. You won't squander time or energy if you lose sight of what has to be done and when.

Deterring Distractions

Interruptions can derail an otherwise productive day. Allowing someone to enter your office to "fast run things by you" can cost you valuable hours of your time. Try these strategies to reduce distractions and keep your day on track.

Set a limit for yourself. When dealing with an interrupter, be strong and tell her right away that your time is valuable. Begin the conversation with a firm "I only have five minutes." "How can I best assist you?" Put a clock on or above your desk to make the time restriction obvious. If the interrupter offers to phone you later, politely decline and say, "No, I'll be busy later." "How can I assist you right now?"

Clear signals should be sent. When the meeting's time limit has passed, shuffle papers on your desk, rise, or use another body language to signal that it is over. You can cushion the impact by keeping a friendly attitude and injecting some humour ("Well, I best get back to this project before the paperwork starts to multiply")- or you can just say thank you, which formally ends the dialogue.

Make your first move. Another approach to conclude a meeting is to inform the interrupter that you have other obligations by asking him to wait a moment while you make a note regarding whatever you're working on. He should eventually get the hint. If nothing else works, break up a long conversation with a surprised, "Wait, what time is it?" It will undoubtedly end the conversation.

Don't wait till tomorrow... Procrastination may derail even the best-laid plans and turn them into a complete disaster. If you have a habit of procrastinating on large or challenging jobs, the tips below might help you modify your habits.

Get it out of the way. When the sequence in which you undertake activities or components of a task is up to you, prioritise the tasks that appear to be the most disagreeable.

That offers you something to look forward to since you know there will be more pleasurable activities ahead. If you do the opposite—take care of what you enjoy first and save what you don't like until later—you're more likely to delay.

Clear the table. If you're having trouble getting started, consider eliminating everything from your desk's surface except items related to the work at hand. The fewer visual distractions you have, the more likely it is that you will be able to focus on what you need to perform.

Find a cheerleader. A coworker can assist you in getting over the procrastination hump by giving you a pre-project pep talk. Find a trailblazer—someone who has already completed the task at hand.

Sneak a preview. If you have a project due on Monday, you should review it the Friday before. When you return to the workplace after the weekend, you will have some sort of familiarity with the project's specifics. This technique also works before you go on vacation—or, for that matter, every time a few days or even a few hours pass before you can start working.

Take little steps. It's quite tempting to put off a major project. Procrastination simply complicates the job—and your life. Instead, break the bi-project into mini-projects and work on each one separately, advises Alan Lakein, a time management consultant to Fortune 500 organisations and author of How to Manage Your Time.

Take back control of your time and life. The project will appear less frightening if you apply this strategy, which Lakein refers to as the Swiss cheese method since it punches holes in cumbersome jobs.

Please make a note of it for the record. When you write down what you're going to do and when you're going to do it, you minimise your chances of delaying. Sharing your deadlines with others can assist even more because it removes any self-imposed hurdles to getting started on time and offers you outside support.

Give yourself some time. When it comes to many projects, you'll want to see it through to completion once you get started. Because you've run out of time, you won't want to pack everything. Start early in the morning, on a day when you don't have anything else planned. That way, you may commit as much time as the assignment necessitates. If you have the option of doing your job in one day, you will most likely do so. Just be sure to take breaks from time to time, so the task doesn't feel too strenuous.

Keep the final goal in mind. Much of what you need to do to attain your goal may not be enjoyable while you're doing it. Finding methods to decrease expenses in your department, for example, so that you're saving more and spending less, won't always make you feel better. When your department gets recognised for performing the best work on the shortest budget, you'll understand that your efforts, as challenging as they were, resulted in a highly gratifying end.

Give yourself a pat on the back for a job well done. If you expect your project to last several days, weeks, or even months, reward yourself whenever you achieve a deadline or finish particularly tough work. Treat yourself to a movie, a massage, or a lunch at your favourite restaurant—whatever you want. These reinforcements might help you stay motivated during the process.

Getting The Most Out Of Meetings

Work might feel like a series of meetings on certain days. You don't have time to attend to your priorities. Meetings are only required for discussing ideas and achieving agreements. Other conversations can be addressed over the phone or by e-mail.

Maintain a schedule and remain within your time constraints. When you need to call a meeting, being prepared allows you to keep it brief and to the point. The following techniques can also be beneficial.

Make a written record of it. Take notes during meetings or delegate this task to someone else. This way, you'll have an exact record of what's been achieved and what still has to be done. Make attendees feel at ease. Find innovative methods to engage and invigorate attendees during potentially dull sessions. Meeting leaders should crack jokes, blow bubbles, and even act outright ridiculously, according to author Steve Kaye in his book.

Meetings that last an hour or less. This calms the participants and helps them to feel at ease, offering even outlandish ideas.

Make your mission more dramatic. Calculate how much the meeting will cost each minute to encourage participants in your meeting to make the most of their time together.

Include the time of the participants, the time of the facilitator, any supplies that will be needed, and so on. Then, at the start of the meeting, remark, "It costs us £100 per minute to be here today, so I propose we make the most use of our time."

Conclusion

Everyone has different motivations for adopting a minimalist life-style. Perhaps you bought this book because your drawers are full, your rooms are untidy, and your closets overflow. Maybe you discovered that going to the shops and buying new stuff isn't making you happy. Perhaps you are concerned about the environmental impact of your consumption, and you are afraid that your children and grandchildren will not have access to the clean air and water that should be their birthright.

I hope the tips on these pages have encouraged you to declutter your house, simplify your life, and live a bit more lightly on the earth. It's a message you won't frequently hear in our "more is better" culture; in fact, you'll nearly always hear the opposite. Commercials, magazines, billboards, radio, and advertisements on buses, benches, buildings, toilet stalls, and even in our schools push us to consume. This is because traditional media channels are primarily controlled by people who profit when we buy more things.

It might feel like you're swimming upstream when you live a simple lifestyle. People who feel threatened by any divergence from the current quo will tell you that you can't possibly live without a vehicle, a television, or a full suite of living room furnishings. They'll tell you that if you don't buy designer clothing, the newest technological devices, and the largest house you can afford, you're not successful. They could even accuse you of being disloyal and a threat to the national economy if you don't spend to your full potential.

Don't trust a word of it. We all know that consumer goods have little to do with life quality and that "stuff" is not a measure of success. A sustainable economy offers far-reaching benefits over an unfettered growth economy, and you can support your nation far more effectively by engaging in community and civic activities than by buying at the shops.

And don't worry, you're not in this alone. Following the recent economic excesses, there is rising dissatisfaction with consumerism and a wave of desire to live simpler, more meaningful lives. Look outside "big media," and you'll discover lots of like-minded people. If you casually mention to a coworker or neighbour that you're "downsizing your things," you'll almost certainly be received with a knowing sigh and a remark along the lines of "I'd like to do that, too."

The Internet, in particular, offers a wealth of knowledge and assistance. The number of blogs and websites advocating minimalist living, voluntary simplicity, and alternative lifestyle design has grown dramatically in recent years. Whether you're looking for tips on clearing out your closets, wondering what it's like to disconnect the TV, or fantasising about selling everything and living out of a suit-case, you'll discover people who have been there, done that, and are willing to share their knowledge. Consider joining a minimalist discussion forum; it's a fantastic opportunity to interact with other minimalists, share decluttering ideas, and get inspiration and encouragement to keep going.

You'll have a fantastic feeling of peace and serenity after you've gone beyond the status quo. When you ignore ads and limit your consumption, there is no cause to yearn for goods, no pressure to acquire them, and no financial strain to pay for them. It's like waving a magic wand and magically removing a slew of concerns and difficulties from your life. You don't care about the "it" hand-bag, the latest vehicle models, or the latest trend in kitchen cabinets

—much less want to work longer hours or max out your credit cards to get them.

Simplicity living brings freedom—liberation from debt, clutter, and the rat race. Each needless object you get rid of in your life— whether it's an underused item, an unnecessary purchase, or an unfulfilling task—feels like a weight off your shoulders. You'll have fewer errands to run, as well as fewer things to buy, pay for, clean, maintain, and insure. You'll feel liberated and fancy-free, ready to go on a dime and chase chances without fretting over your belongings. Furthermore, when you aren't chasing status symbols or keeping up with the Joneses, you have more time and energy for more satisfying activities, such as playing with your children, volunteering in your community, and contemplating the purpose of life.

This freedom, in turn, provides a fantastic chance for self-discovery. We lose our sense of self when we identify with brands and express ourselves via material possessions. We utilise consumer goods to project a particular image of ourselves to the rest of the world— buying a character to display the rest of the world. We begin to see ourselves as the guy who wears Gucci, the lady who adores Tiffany, and the man who drives a Mercedes. Furthermore, we are so preoccupied with things—running to and fro, purchasing this and that—that we have little time to pause and reflect on what truly makes us tick.

When we become minimalists, we remove all the excess— brands, status symbols, collections, and clutter—to reveal our genuine selves. We take the time to reflect on who we are, what is important to us, and what genuinely makes us happy. We escape from our consumerism cocoons to fly as poets, philosophers, artists, activists, moms, dads, spouses, and friends. Above all, we reinvent ourselves via what we do, how we think, and who we love, rather than through what we acquire.

There's an old Buddhist story about a man who visited a Zen master, seeking spiritual guidance. Instead of listening, the guest focused on his views. After a time, the master brought out tea. He poured into the visitor's cup, then continued to pour till it ran over onto the table. The guest, surprised, shouted that the cup was full— and questioned why he kept pouring when there was no more room!

The instructor emphasised that the guest, like the cup, was already full of his thoughts and opinions—and that he couldn't learn anything until his cup was emptied.

The same thing happens when our lives are overburdened with obligations, clutter, and non-essentials. We don't make "space" for new experiences, and as a result, we miss out on opportunities to grow and deepen our relationships. Becoming minimalists aids us in resolving this. We empty our cups by removing the excess from our homes, schedules, and brains, allowing us the limitless capacity for life, love, hopes, goals, and abundant quantities of joy.

Feedback

Thank you for reading 'Why Living A Simple Life Is Better For You'. We hope you enjoyed the book? Please now scan the QR code below to leave your feedback.

SCAN ME

Claim Your Freebie NOW!

Get Good At Problem Solving

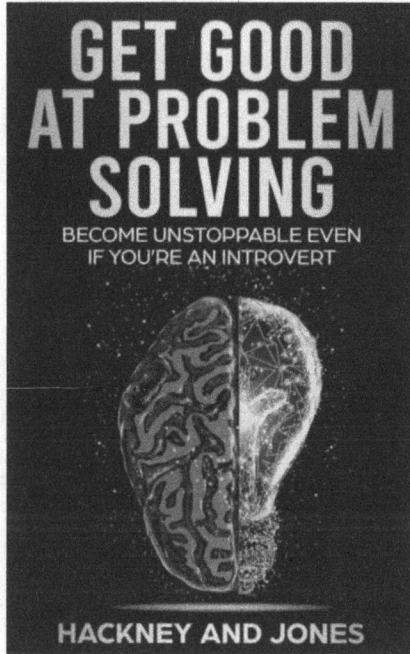

Want to know the secret behind getting good at problem solving? Everyone seems to be able to do it, but you're stuck in the pile of endless to-do lists with little progress.

Ok, so how do I get my FREE book?

EASY! See the next page

Claim Your Freebie NOW

Instructions:

1. Open the camera or the QR reader application on your smartphone.

2. Point your camera at the QR code to scan the QR code.

3. A notification will pop-up on screen.

4. Click on the notification to open the website link

SCAN ME

Also By Rachel Stone

How To Remove Negativity From Your Life

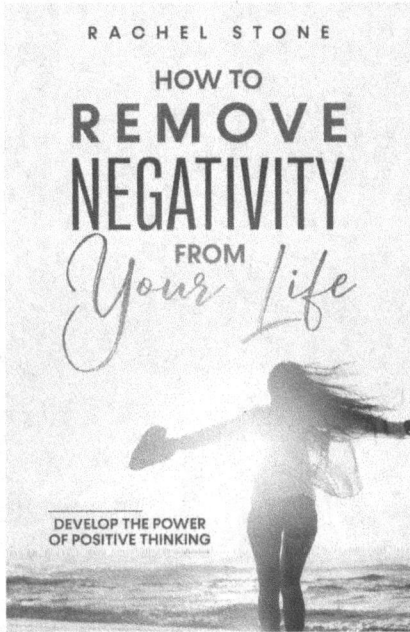

RACHEL STONE

HOW TO
REMOVE
NEGATIVITY
FROM
Your Life

DEVELOP THE POWER
OF POSITIVE THINKING

Rid yourself forever from the negative thoughts that
plague your life with this amazing, life-changing book.

Also By Rachel Stone

Start Being Fearless, Stop Being Scared

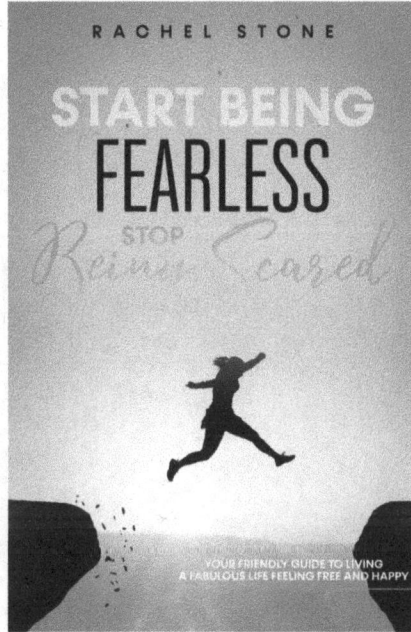

Fed up of being scared of the things in life that hold you back? It's time to take control back and start being fearless.

Also By Rachel Stone

How To Heal Toxic Thoughts

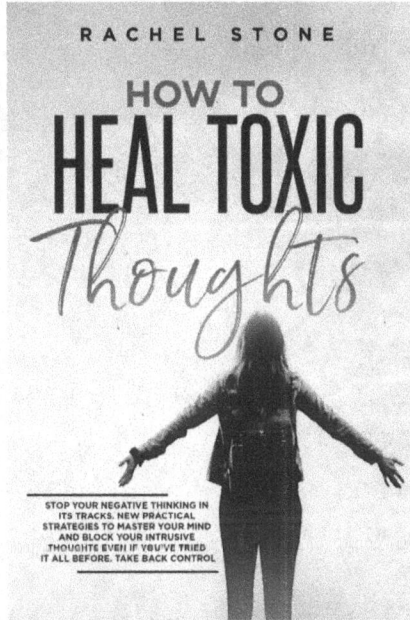

Are you sick of your whole day being ruined due to your overthinking? Have you had enough of self-sabotaging everything good in your life? Do you want practical strategies to finally have a peaceful night's sleep?

Grab the Rachel Stone series NOW

Instructions:

1. Open the camera or the QR reader application on your smartphone.

2. Point your camera at the QR code to scan the QR code.

3. A notification will pop-up on screen.

4. Click on the notification to open the website link

SCAN ME